The New Basic Anti-Inflammatory Diet

An Easy and Quick Guide for a Natural and Healthy Lifestyle to Decrease Inflammation Level in Human Body and Finally Live Pain-Free Based on the Latest Studies and Evidences

By Susan Sanderson

This eBook is provided with the sole purpose of providing relevant information on a specific topic for which every reasonable effort has been made to ensure that it is both accurate and reasonable. Nevertheless, by purchasing this eBook you consent to the fact that the author, as well as the publisher, are in no way experts on the topics contained herein, regardless of any claims as such that may be made within. As such, any suggestions or recommendations that are made within are done so purely for entertainment value. It is recommended that you always consult a professional prior to undertaking any of the advice or techniques discussed within.

This is a legally binding declaration that is considered both valid and fair by both the Committee of Publishers Association and the American Bar Association and should be considered as legally binding within the United States.

The reproduction, transmission, and duplication of any of the content found herein, including any specific or extended information will be done as an illegal act regardless of the end form the information ultimately takes. This includes copied versions of the work both physical, digital and audio unless express consent of the Publisher is provided beforehand. Any additional rights reserved.

Furthermore, the information that can be found within the pages described forthwith shall be considered both accurate and truthful when it comes to the recounting of facts. As such, any use, correct or incorrect, of the provided information will render the Publisher free of responsibility as to the actions taken outside of their direct purview. Regardless, there are zero scenarios where the original author or the Publisher can be deemed liable in any fashion for any damages or hardships that may result from any of the information discussed herein.

Additionally, the information in the following pages is intended only for informational purposes and should thus be thought of as universal. As befitting its nature, it is presented without assurance regarding its prolonged validity or interim quality. Trademarks that are mentioned are done without written consent and can in no way be considered an endorsement from the trademark holder.

Table of Contents

Introduction

You just did something good for yourself by selecting this copy of *The New Basic Anti-Inflammatory Diet*. You should be proud! You will feel truly fortunate that you came across this new approach to getting the level of health people strive for using various other methods, yet often don't achieve.

What is inflammation? When our bodies perceive a threat to our health, it produces chemicals and white blood cells to combat bacteria, viruses and infection. Sometimes the body's immune system will work overtime when dealing with various autoimmune diseases. Crohn's disease, celiac disease, fibromyalgia, multiple sclerosis, and even osteoarthritis can trigger an inflammatory response when no imminent threat is present. Inflammation, in the forms of infections, high blood pressure, painful joints, can even promote the development of abnormal cell growth, i.e., cancer cells.

Through nutrition, supplements, herbs, exercise and a return to nature, these inflammatory responses can be reduced or eliminated. From this plan, one can enjoy more energy, weight loss, a reduction in blood pressure, better sleep, less joint and muscle pain and ease from various autoimmune diseases. Results are usually noticeable very quickly.

This book includes lifestyle suggestions, lists of foods and herbs that you will immediately recognize and be able to find in almost all grocery stores. Simple meal ideas have been included to help you get a foothold on getting started with this new way to approach nutrition and health.

Begin your journey confident that this strategy is one you will be thrilled with and will want to share with family and friends!

Chapter 1: What Inflammation Is and What Is it Doing to You?

Inflammation is your friend. You've heard that, right? It's trying to help you out. Well, yes, most of the time it is.

When your body detects harm, it tries to fight for you. It tries to fix or remove the problem. Your body is attempting to heal itself. It's called the "immune response." For example: You cut or bump your knee. Your body sends a flood of white blood cells to the area. You'll see swelling, redness (your knee will probably look blue and purple pretty quickly). If you don't see these things, it means that your immune system is on the snooze for some reason. That's not good. But we normally do see these things and this response says that you're on the way to healing yourself. This is a good thing, of course. This is called an "acute" response.

However, a "chronic" response is due to on-going sustained, unwanted substances and conditions within the body. Exposure to cigarette smoke and the storage of excess fat cells can bring on some serious issues. You might be seeing a little tire around your middle. It's from fat cells lodging there. Unfortunately, these fat cells can then lodge inside your arteries causing atherosclerosis. An alarm goes off inside your body and it sends a team of white cells to the rescue. And it can send these "rescuers" over and over. These sticky cells attach themselves to the fat cells, then mix it up with blood cells and can erupt the arteries. Lots of times they can cause blockage, at the least, and voila! You've set yourself up for a stroke or heart attack. There is a plethora of other health issues and conditions related to chronic inflammation. This is what this book is about.

You can have your doctor check to see if this chronic inflammation is happening or not. There is this simple blood test called hsCRP that measures the C-reactive protein (a bio-marker for inflammation). It reports if there is any arterial inflammation. If your score is high, and you're a male, Harvard found out about 20 years ago that you'll be three times as likely to experience a heart attack, and twice as prone to having a stroke as the rest of the non-inflamed (or less-inflamed) population. But, (a disclaimer here), your inflammation score doesn't need to be all that high to bring on these dire health concerns.

Some doctors prescribe statins, along with some lifestyle changes. We'll get to those lifestyle modifications very soon and see if things can be brought back to a healthy level in order to avoid medication.

How do you know if you've got a problem with inflammation? Here are some signals you might want to pay attention to.

Are you having problems losing those extra pounds and keeping them off? Has your doctor told you that you're diabetic? That's a clue that inflammation has set up shop in your immune system. You might be carrying a lot of visceral fat. This is the fat that surrounds internal organs. It's very difficult to get rid of.

Belly cramping, digestive problems, gut pain and diarrhea are indicative of inflammatory bowel disease. If you've already been diagnosed with ulcerative colitis or Crohn's disease, those are very much connected to inflammatory disease.

Osteoarthritis, also aggravated by inflammation, is one thing. That happens when cartilage breaks down as we age, and we experience joint pain that is generally manageable. But, rheumatoid arthritis, RA, is another creature. This is when the inflammation aggressively attacks joints in a way that prevents any repair. You'll be visited by intense pain, stiff, red, warm and swollen joints tender to the touch. It makes it very difficult to move. Harm from RA can also damage the heart.

More recent research suggests that brain inflammation is a strong connection to fibromyalgia. It doesn't affect the joints. This type of inflammation creates painful muscle sensitivity and exhaustion. Fibromyalgia continues to be studied, but inflammation appears to be the culprit.

Sometimes symptoms can present loudly and quickly. Other times, it progresses slowly and quietly. Alzheimer's is being researched with a focus on inflammation being the cause. Studies are being conducted on whether an anti-inflammatory diet can stave off or prevent this dreadful disease.

Diet matters. We're hearing more about "plant-based" diets. Good for us, good for the planet. We're reminded to eat our "colors." Put plenty of fruits and vegetables in your shopping cart, on your plate, and eat them! Include whole grains, certain animal proteins, legumes and foods with omega-e fatty acids in your diet. Use healthier cooking oils and make sure to get foods that contain probiotics. Cut out saturated fats and watch the sugar!

How can this happen, you ask? Read on, friend! There is a lot to learn.

Chapter 2: Food and Inflammation. How What You Eat Affects Your Body

"You are what you eat." We've heard that quip for a long time. The first time anybody used that saying was back in 1826, coined by Anthelme Brillat-Savarin in his book *Physiologie du Gout*. (It's got a really long title. I'll spare you that detail!) But it is absolutely true.

There are so many foods that are good for you, but this chapter isn't about them. This chapter is about the stuff we love, but are truly "no-no's" as a regular diet choice for people who want or need to reduce the inflammation in their systems. Let's look at them. You'll soon see why we need to keep a watch on these foods.

Sugar and High Fructose Corn Syrup

Pies, cakes, candy bars, sodas, fruit juices are on this highly recognizable list. These treats, and other foods, have something in common, and you guessed it. Sugar. Processed sugar, aka sucrose, glucose or fructose. Sugar has lots of names, 56 of them, in fact. Here are a few that you'll know: brown sugar, beet sugar, cane juice, cane sugar, corn syrup, confectioner's sugar, dextrose, honey, lactose and malt. If you look at labels on processed foods, you'll see many of these listed. Any sugar we ingest with a name that ends with "ose" tells our bodies to release cytokines.

The job of cytokines is that of a messenger. These protein molecules assist in cell communication telling other cells to gather at a sight of infection, trauma and inflammation.

Sweet, sugary drinks like sodas, are loaded with fructose. We don't feel satisfied when we consume fructose, so then it's easy to follow up by consuming a high number of calories through multiple sugary drinks trying to quench our thirst and our craving for something sweet. Research has consistently shown that people who drink sugary beverages are more overweight than those who do not. These same people are found to have more visceral fat. That fat that is found deep in the body. It surrounds organs. Visceral fat contributes to heart disease and diabetes. It's the most difficult fat to get rid of and the most dangerous to carry around.

Fructose, more than glucose, is what makes you think you want more. Excessive fructose decreases the hormone leptin. Leptin's job is to tell your body that you feel full; that you don't need anything more to eat or drink. If that is impaired, you never know when you're feeling full.

Another problem associated with sugary drinks is the link to atherosclerosis, a disease that clogs arteries with fatty deposits called arterial plaque. This plaque is made up of calcium, cholesterol, cellular waste and something called fibrin. Fibrin promotes blood clotting. Your immune system complicates things by sending in even more blood cells to continue to clog and block your arteries. When the walls of your arteries become hard and narrow, the condition is called atherosclerosis. Strokes and possible heart attacks can be the result of this disease.

Who loves bread? Who loves pasta and starchy foods, in general? Well, who doesn't? Not to make you sad, but starchy foods contain glucose.

Glucose isn't all bad now. Glucose is what gives our cells the energy to make muscle and soft tissue. It gives our brains the ability to function smoothly. It comes from what we eat, obviously, and is also produced by our liver. Ideally, our livers will produce the right amount of glucose to fuel our cells, but not enough to overwhelm the bloodstream. Our pancreas assists in this to produce the right amount of insulin that transports the glucose from out of our bloodstream to our cells. That's the way it's supposed to work.

On-going high blood sugar levels can develop a condition called hyperglycemia, which means that our pancreas isn't producing enough insulin. A lack of insulin, or none at all, compels glucose to dump into the blood stream instead of feeding cells. And that situation is prime for developing diabetes.

Diets that contain a high amount of refined carbohydrates promote all kinds of problems, including acne and prematurely aging skin. Foods with a high glycemic index (processed, sweet foods) raise your blood sugar more quickly than foods with low glycemic indexes. The rapid spikes and drops in blood sugar and insulin levels increase androgen secretion, oil production and inflammation resulting in acne. It's been found that people who live in rural areas, who are eating more foods that aren't highly processed and "improved" with sugars, have a much lower incidence of acne.

A diet high in sugar speeds up the appearance of wrinkles and loose skin. AGEs, advanced glycation end products, are created by the interaction of sugar with protein. These AGEs damage collagen and elastin. The skin no longer looks youthful and fresh. A diet of low carbs, restricted sugar and protein is what you need as you age to preserve great skin.

The strongest risk factor in the development of diabetes is obesity. The consumption of sugar in drinks and foods is a primary cause of weight gain. The long-term consumption of sugar can also lead to insulin resistance. Blood sugar levels rise and diabetes develops when people become insulin resistant.

It's fun to treat ourselves to pastries, muffins, and have the occasional splurge at a fast food restaurant. But if these indulgences become the norm, we can get in big trouble. The documented increased cancer risk from additional sugar consumption needs to be recognized. The ingredients used to put together these treats are comprised of refined carbohydrates. Almost all of the fiber has been removed, stripping these foods of any beneficial nutrition. Fiber is necessary to improve the good bacteria that resides in your gut. It also makes us feel full and boosts blood sugar control. Women who consume cookies and pastries three times a week, have been identified to be almost 1.5 times more likely to develop endometrial cancer than those females who splurge only .5 times a week. (It's puzzling as to how a person can go out a half a time a week to get a beignet, but researchers seem to know how to do this. Statistics!)

Another study of 430,000 people found that the risk of developing esophageal cancer, pleural cancer, and cancer of the small intestine was associated with the increased consumption of sugar.

Beating the "Blues" with a sugary delight, only makes the depression worse. The blood sugar swings, inflammation from these processed foods, and neurotransmitter dysregulation creates an environment in your brain conducive to experiencing increased bouts of depression. Ironically, processed foods that tout being "low fat" luring you to think you are doing something positive for yourself, boost the flavor of the food with even more sugar. It's a lose-lose situation. So frustrating. Again, read your labels.

Curbing Sugar Cravings

There are ways to curb sugar cravings. Start by making sure that you are eating an appropriate amount of protein. It will cut the craving for sugar. Aside from managing the hunger for sweets, protein assists with the digestive process. Protein builds muscle and connective tissues and protects the nervous system. Vegetarians and vegans can build up protein reserves by consuming legumes, non-GMO tofu, seeds, nuts and beans.

Drinking water before mealtime helps you to feel full. This will contribute to weight loss and will stave off the interest in having dessert.

Getting a good night's sleep reduces the hormone ghrelin aka the "hunger hormone." When you're deprived to sleep, thoughts of convenience foods and sugary foods activate the pleasure center of the brain often leading people to make poor choices. Giving yourself 7-8 hours of sleep can reduce sugar cravings.

Having a "cuppa" tea has been found to reduce the yearn for a sugary treat. Adding cinnamon, ginger and turmeric to hot drinks will balance your blood sugar levels and curb the craving for something sweet. Add a healthy fat to tea to make it even more satisfying. Coconut milk or ghee will also contribute to the balance of blood sugar.

Serve yourself more chromium rich foods. Broccoli, romaine lettuce, asparagus, oats, prunes, green beans, and mushrooms are good suppliers of chromium. These foods soothe the urge to consume sugar. Chromium reduces the feeling of being hungry, promotes weight loss, improves blood glucose levels in diabetics and lowers the risk of type 2 diabetes.

Switch to alternative sugars such as honey, maple syrup, Stevia, or coconut sugar. These sweeteners are a better choice because they have a wealth of vitamins, minerals, and are a source of antioxidants. These choices are a good way to dodge consumption of sugar.

While at the store, don't put sugary treats in your shopping cart. Don't bring them home. Turn to fruit, vegetables, nuts, seeds and gluten-free grains when the itch for sugar strikes.

Preservatives and Additives

Another inflammatory ingredient found in many processed foods are additives. Lots of times, we don't even think about them. They are added to our foods, many times condiments and practically all processed foods, to improve appearance, enhance flavor, extend shelf-life, give vivid color, and fight mold. Let's examine what these additives can potentially do to you.

Look in your refrigerator and check the labels on condiments. This is a list of what you'll find in terms of preservatives and additives: ascorbic acid, calcium chloride, calcium disodium, sodium benzoate, sodium nitrite (found in processed meats), sulfur dioxide, potassium chloride, potassium sorbate, polysorbate 60, tocopherols, and xanthan gum. Remember, this is only a partial list of those additives that are fairly familiar. All of these are probably familiar to you.

A little more on sodium benzoate that was just mentioned above. This is an additive that you'll find in sodas, salad dressings, pickles and many condiments. Here are some of the concerns raised by researchers. One study found that university students that consumed a greater amount of beverages that contained sodium benzoate had more symptoms of ADHD. Combining sodium benzoate with vitamin C, which then converts to benzene, appears to have a link to certain cancers. Sugar-free carbonated drinks contain high levels of benzene. Other carbonated beverages also contain benzene. Another study connected hyperactivity in 3 year-olds exposed to foods that had a combination of sodium benzoate and artificial food coloring. The general consensus is to make a real effort to avoid foods that combine sodium benzoate and vitamin C, (benzene), a compound found to be cancer causing.

The food color, Red 40 (which replaced Red 3 several years ago), is still regarded as a possible culprit for shorter attention spans and hyperactivity in children. These days, food coloring is primarily made from petroleum products. Certain dyes contribute to cancer.

Nitrites, found in bacon, ham, sausage and processed lunch meats, when exposed to heat and amino acids turn into nitrosamine, which has been linked to colorectal cancer. So, please limit putting these meats on your plate.

Artificial Sweeteners

Artificial sweeteners have a checkered reputation. They are used for assisting in weight loss. And they help without too much harm according to what the medical world knows about them right now. However, there is a school of thought that they are probably cancer producing. Moderate use is the key. Some people are sensitive to these substances and develop headaches. These sweeteners are found to not raise blood pressure by themselves, but the catch to using artificial sweeteners is that they are combined with other foods and ingredients that can be inflammatory. For example, that chocolate bar you love that's sweetened with aspartame also has caffeine and processed fats which are inflammatory substances, and contain calories.

Two out of five Americans consume artificial sweeteners on a regular basis. Many artificial sweeteners have not been approved for use in numerous other countries. Some of the concerns are that they block the "food reward pathway," interfering with leptin's job of telling you that you're feeling full. Since the molecules are very similar to regular sugar, but lack the calories, these sweeteners trick the brain into thinking it needs more food, and so, we eat more. Some researchers are finding that artificial sweeteners actually create cravings for more sweet food. The cravings are then satisfied by consuming even more artificially sweet foods with refined carbohydrate content thereby creating inflammation.

Here are few sweetener names that you'll probably know: Equal, NutraSweet, Splenda, Sugar Twin, Sweet n Low. Use them in moderation.

Sugar alcohols, another artificial sweetener, are found naturally in fruits and vegetables and are also made chemically. These are not alcohols that will get you tipsy, by the way. This substance isn't processed by the body the way regular sugar is. It's not fully absorbed during digestion, and so it delivers half the calories that sugar does. Even though its impact on blood sugar is less than regular sugar, it is still a carbohydrate and can affect blood sugar levels if consumed too often. As a diabetic, one may confuse the idea that sugar alcohols provide fewer calories, and so it's okay to consume more calories. It's good to keep in mind that the rest of the foods and drinks do contain other carbohydrates that can influence blood sugar levels and trigger inflammation.

Sugar and Telomeres

Our genetic information is found inside the nucleus of our cells. This information is arranged on the twisted strands of molecules called DNA. This contains all of our genetic data. Capping and protecting these chromosomes are other chromosomes, called telomeres that guard this genetic information and make it possible for these chromosomes to do their work properly. Telomeres prevent the DNA strands from tangling and fusing together and protect the genetic information within the DNA. Higher levels of sugar consumption accelerate the degeneration of the telomeres and then our chromosomes begin to shorten, which promotes cellular aging. This early aging is a primary risk factor for cancer, diabetes, cardio-vascular disease and neurodegenerative disorders.

Research corroborates that destruction of telomeres is a major cause of aging and more rapid decline. Here is a list of age-related diseases related to telomere damage due to substantial sugar consumption: renal dysfunction, type 2 diabetes, fibrosis, non-alcoholic fatty liver disease, cardiovascular disease, osteoarthritis, general decline in immune function, sarcopenia, and age-related wastage (cachexia).

Beyond the diseases already listed from too much sugar are other conditions that impact health. Poor dental health, impaired memory, cognitive decline, dementia.

These conditions and diseases are all caused by high levels of sugar consumption and inflammation. Extra sugar must be kept to a minimum. The inflammation caused by it has too many negative consequences.

Trans-fats and Saturated Fats

Trans-fats are widely recognized to be responsible for numerous health issues. Since June 2, 2018, they have been officially banned from the United States. Trans fats were produced by a process that pumps hydrogen molecules along with hydrogen gas and metallic catalysts into vegetable oils. This process is called hydrogenation. It extends the shelf-life of foods. Vegetable shortening, some brands of microwave popcorn, margarine, non-dairy coffee creamers, frozen pizza, canned frosting, ice cream, pudding, potato chips and corn chips have long been guilty of high trans-fat content. Now they are guilty of having a high saturated fat content. Many manufacturers have now become informed and cautious about high levels of trans-fats and saturated fats and have reduced the amount used in their production of food. Fried fast foods is another thing. The heat required to cook these foods with higher levels of these fats, increase the fat content which is effused into the food being cooked.

Trans-fats also occur naturally in foods from ruminant animals, cattle, sheep and goats (think red meat, cheeses, dairy products). The ruminant trans fats are created in the animals' gut while digesting grass. Do not be alarmed. These foods can be eaten, of course in moderation. One ruminant trans-fat is CLA, conjugated linoleic acid, which is often used as a weight loss supplement.

In the past thirty years, there have been multiple studies on artificially made trans- fats wherein test subjects were evaluated on risk factors for heart disease and cholesterol counts. It was consistently found that with the ingestion of trans-fats, LDL levels, the bad cholesterol, rose significantly. HDL was lowered by consuming trans-fats. Trans-fats damage the interior lining, the endothelium, of arteries. Clinical trials and observational studies conclude that the consumption of trans-fats was an aggressive contributor of heart disease and stroke. Eating trans-fats and saturated fats also contribute to the risk of type 2 diabetes, and breast cancer in women.

The FDA has now determined that trans-fats from partially hydrogenated vegetable oils can no longer be "generally recognized as safe." And be aware that palm oils and coconut oils contain a lot of saturated fat. This fat also raises your total cholesterol. Twenty to thirty-five percent of your total daily calories can come from fat. But only 10% of total daily calories should be from saturated fat.

Ways to reduce the chance of encountering saturated fats would be to:
~Limit the consumption of commercially prepared baked goods and fried foods.
~Use soft margarine instead of stick margarine, if you're going to use any at all.
~Cook with non-hydrogenated oils such as safflower oil, sunflower oil, canola oil using extra virgin olive oil most often.
~Avoid commercially prepared foods such as pies, cakes, muffins, crackers, cookies and donuts often are made with saturated fat.
~Stick to a dietary plan that emphasizes fruits, vegetables, whole grains, lean protein, fatty fish, poultry and nuts.
~Prepare your own food and eat at home more often.
Note that monounsaturated fat from olive oil, peanut and canola oil are much healthier choices than saturated fats.

Chapter 3: Role of Sleep as Part of the Anti-Inflammatory Approach to Health

The majority of studies on sleep have focused on the quantity of sleep. More time is now being spent on researching and identifying the quality of sleep. A publication in the journal, *Geriatric & Gerontology International*, reported results of a study of 1,639 adults age 65 and older. The study was based on a survey about the quality of sleep, sleep habits, sleep disruption patterns, difficulty or ease of falling asleep and diet. It was shown that people who followed a Mediterranean style diet (an anti-inflammation diet) proved to have the better sleep experiences.

Mary Yannakoulia, PhD, Department of Nutrition and Dietetics at Harokopio University, Athens, Greece reported that "...the Mediterranean diet was not significantly related to sleep duration. In fact, sleep quality is viewed as a more complete index making it the most important sleep measure associated with dietary choices."

The foods found in the Mediterranean diet, fruits, vegetables, nuts, certain kinds of fish, olive oil are great sources of melatonin. This is a neurohormone that regulates circadian rhythms which impacts the sleep-wake cycle by promoting sleep. Of course, we can find melatonin tablets on the shelf at the grocery store, but we'd be cheating ourselves out of the other positive benefits of an anti-inflammatory diet.

Quality sleep is important for many reasons. One is that it protects your heart. Sleep disorders have been linked to cardio-vascular diseases. Not getting enough sleep promotes weight gain. Lack of sleep changes the way our bodies store and use carbohydrates and alters the amount of hormones that affect our appetite.

Sleep deprivation changes our immune system. It affects how the killer cells function. The lack of quality sleep has been linked to cancer. Researchers have found that melatonin levels are affected by light exposure. People who do shift work often complain of sleep disorders. Melatonin protects us against developing cancer tumors. Even light from nightlights and electronics can affect how our body produces this hormone. Our sleeping space should be as dark as possible.

A good night's sleep helps our memory and the way we think, learn and solve problems. Sleeping well keeps us alert during the day.

Good sleep reduces stress. When w are stressed, we produce a hormone called cortisol. Cortisol is directly linked to high blood pressure, weight gain and ultimately diabetes.

Catching our "zzzz's" protects our health in so many other ways. Sleep studies have shown reduction in depression for test subjects. Other research has tied quality sleep to intentional weight loss, better moods, and reduction in accidents. Sleep is important for our bodies to heal from sickness, and injury. Sleep repairs damage from ultraviolet rays, stress, and harmful exposure from elements in the environment.

Quality sleep is as important as food, exercise and relaxation. You will soon see how these elements work together to protect your body from disease and to promote health.

Chapter 4: What Foods are Anti-Inflammatory?

As will be further discussed in Chapter 5, you'll see how stress, lack of sleep, and a sedate lifestyle can exacerbate inflammation. This can be combated with foods that promote healing. This is not to say to allow stress to engulf your life and spend free time in front of a television or a computer. But healthy, anti-inflammatory food choices certainly do so much to improve blood sugar levels and support your body's system of protection from everything from colds to cancer.

Fruit

Let's begin with fruit. Fruit is sweet and refreshing. It's a treat by itself and can be added to so many recipes. It does contain carbohydrates, but these are complex carbohydrates. Simple or refined carbohydrates are digested quickly, flood your blood stream with sugar, and move through your system stripped of nutrients, minerals, and fiber. They create inflammation, weight gain and disease.

Complex carbohydrates, on the other hand, are quite different. These flood your system with vitamins, minerals, and fiber. They digest more slowly and so raise blood sugars in a slower, more controlled way. Fruit is an example of a complex carbohydrate. Complex carbohydrates from berries contain anti-oxidants called anthocyanins. These reduce inflammation, support our immune system, and reduce risk of heart disease.

Oxidative stress occurs when the number of free radicals, which are unstable molecules, gets too high. Oxidative stress accelerates cell and tissue damage which is at the beginning of the road to cancer, heart disease, and diabetes.

Multiple studies have shown the positive effects of adding anti-oxidants from berries in diets. They work fighting free radicals. The berries with the most anti-radicals are blueberries, black berries, raspberries, and pomegranates. However, other berries can offer enormous health benefits, too.

One study showed that a group of healthy people who consumed 17 ounces of strawberry pulp for thirty days reduced their pro-oxidant markers by 30%.
Another study that demonstrated reduction of oxidative stress by eating berries was conducted with a group of healthy, adult males. They managed to protect their DNA against free radical damage by merely consuming only one 10 ounce serving of blueberries.

Healthy People 2020, is a science-based on-line publication that has established goals to empower the public to make informed, healthy choices and study the impact of prevention strategies. This group of researchers are advising the American public to up their intake of fruit and vegetables to 75%, which equates to two plus servings of fruit per day.

All berries are a great source of polyphenols, which protect the body's tissues against oxidative stress and associated diseases such as cancer, coronary heart disease and other diseases created by inflammation. They are high in providing moisture and are low in calories.

Cherries

After exercising, eat a handful of tart or sweet cherries to ease muscle pain. Cherries are found to reduce the pain of osteo-arthritis. One study has shown that these cherries have the highest anti-oxidant count of any fruit. They contain polyphenols and vitamin C that reduce inflammation and oxidative stress. Tart cherries were identified to have the most polyphenol compounds, which protect body tissues and fight pathologies such as cancers and coronary heart disease. Sweet cherries are found to provide the most anthocyanins that contain anti-oxidant effects. Numerous studies cite that the consumption of cherries improves cardio-vascular health, non-alcoholic liver disease, metabolic syndrome and diabetes to name a few.

Avocados

Another fruit that has seen lots of popularity in bowls of guacamole is the avocado. They are linked to reducing cancer risk because they contain magnesium, potassium, monounsaturated fats, and the very important by-product, fiber.

Avocados have more potassium than a banana. They provide more protein than any other fruit. They have 4 grams of protein. Avocados have 18 of all the important amino acids. The amino acids, anti-oxidants and essential oils can repair damaged hair, soothe burns, and improve skin texture.

Grapes

One of the best sources of resveratrol are grapes. Resveratrol supports brain function, lowers blood pressure and prevents chronic diseases. Resveratrol is the compound found primarily in the skin of red grapes. It has been identified as reducing the risk of atherosclerosis (inflammation and hardening of the arteries), cardio-vascular disease and reduction in blood pressure.

Grapes also contain anthocyanins that reduce inflammation. They provide moisture for our skin and tissues. Just one cup of grapes contains over 120 grams of water. Another anti-inflammatory found in grapes is quercetin that reportedly prevents or can slow growth of cancer cells.

Eaten alone or added to other dishes, grapes are a delicious food source that will enhance your overall health.

Green Leafy Vegetables

Popeye knew what he was doing every time he opened a can of spinach and swallowed it down! He knew that this dark, green leafy vegetable would provide him with vitamins A, D, E, and K which all fight inflammation. Most green leafy vegetables contain alpha-linolenic acid, which is an omega-3 fat that is beneficial with its anti-inflammatory properties. Green, leafy vegetables, broccoli and brussels sprouts included, also contain a compound call quercetin. Quercetin fights joint pain the way aspirin and ibuprofen do, but also block the TNF (tumor necrosis factor) that is found in the joints of people who have rheumatoid arthritis. Greens help reduce cholesterol, boost bone health, lessen joint pain, lower blood pressure and balances glucose levels.

Dark, leafy greens, flip the switch on a gene called the T-bet gene. It informs the pre-curser cells in your intestinal lining to generate innate lymphoid cells that protect your body against gut infections and inflammation, controls reactions against food allergies and seals fissures in a leaky gut. If you eat your greens, you'll be protecting yourself against a host of chronic diseases.

Dark, leafy vegetables provide so many vitamins, minerals and amazing nutrients that support the health of our entire system. Greens contain folate that helps your body to generate more dopamine and serotonin, mood stabilizers. Magnesium is linked to vascular health, and a more regular digestive system. The calcium that dark, leafy greens supply would allow a person to discontinue all dairy if that was an objective.

Romaine lettuce fits into this green and leafy category. Chard fits. Arugula is part of this clan. Spinach, of course fits. So do collard greens and kale. So many people still panic when they see these last two. There are ways of preparing kale and collard greens that make them palatable and ready to be included in salads and main and side dishes.

Iceberg lettuce does not fit into this group of vegetables. It doesn't have enough chlorophyll as do the greens listed above to allow it to be included. Because of that, it doesn't provide the vitamins, minerals, phytonutrients that the dark green, leafy vegetables offer.

Lots of the important nutrients in leafy greens can be absorbed more fully when prepared with an oil, preferably extra virgin olive oil. So, don't be afraid to have a salad, for instance, with a full-fat salad dressing. More nutrients are absorbed this way than with a low-fat dressing (which is typically made with additional sugar to enhance the taste because of it being low-fat).

Some leafy greens can release nutrients better when cooked. Others are better for you eaten raw.

A little word of caution. If you have been prescribed a blood thinning medication, do check with your doctor prior to consuming greens that have a high level of vitamin K. It could possibly interfere with blood clotting.

Olive Oil

EVOO, extra virgin olive oil, is one of the best monounsaturated fats you can eat. It's primarily comprised of oleic acid which reduces inflammation and has positive effects on genes that are at risk for cancer. These anti-inflammatory benefits are far more present in the extra virgin olive oil than in other types of olive oils. These benefits include reduced risk of heart disease, brain cancer, protection against stroke, and lowers the risk of type 2 diabetes.

In a large series of studies that involved over 840,000 people, it was found that this fat was the only kind of monounsaturated fat that reduced the incidence of stroke and heart disease. These findings were further supported by another study of 140,000 people who also used extra virgin olive oil.

Extra virgin olive oil can reduce inflammation. A key anti-oxidant, oleocanthal, works as the anti-inflammatory drug, ibuprofen. But there are findings that are even more impressive.

In a recent study, it was determined that oleocanthal can actually kill cancer cells. The results of this study were published in 2015 by the journal *Molecular and Cellular Oncology*.

They found that this ingredient, oleocanthal, ruptures part of the cancer cell releasing enzymes that produce cell death. It doesn't harm healthy cells. Essentially, cancer cells can become responsible for their own death.

This oleocanthal is made when the olives are crushed while being pressed for oil. The researchers confirmed that oleocanthal causes cancer cell death to happen quickly. Within 30 minutes after contact, the cancer cells are broken down and are destroyed, as opposed to programmed cell death which takes 16 to 24 hours to achieve.

Many studies show that oleocanthal obstructs growth of cancer pathways and the development of cancer processes. It's been documented to shrink cancer cells in mice.

Monounsaturated fatty acids (MUFAs) such as olive oil, has been studied to see if it can benefit blood sugar control and insulin levels. Results are indicating that it's particularly useful if you are at risk for type 2 diabetes.

Olive oil is the main source of fat in the Mediterranean diet. Death rates from cardiovascular diseases are reported to be much lower in that region of the world.

Researchers in France are in agreement that olive oil may prevent stroke in the elderly. It was found that older people who regularly used olive oil in their cooking, or for salad dressing or for use as a bread dip were at a lower risk for stroke by 41 percent.

Aside from its beneficial fatty acids, olive oil is nutritious. It provides vitamins E and K and contain anti-oxidants that are biologically active and may reduce your risk for heart disease, and protect your blood cholesterol from oxidation.

Olive is not associated with weight gain. In a 30-month study of 7,000 Spanish college students, no link was found that the consumption of olive oil contributed to any weight gain. And in a three-year study of 187 participants, it was found that the increased levels of anti-oxidants in their blood contributed to weight loss.

Fatty Fish

All fish contain at least some level of omega-3 fatty acids. But this section will be about the benefits of fish and other foods that have the highest content of omega-3s. Fish with high omega-3 levels are the best kinds of fatty fish to eat because they provide more EPA and DPA, which reduce inflammation. Risk of arthritis, diabetes, heart disease, kidney disease, and metabolic syndrome is substantially lessened by consuming fatty fish. Omega-3 fatty acids also check inflammation in the blood vessels.

Omega-3s have a stabilizing effect on the cardio-vascular system preventing abnormal heart rhythms. If you've already had a heart attack, a prescribed dose of omega-3 can help to protect your heart. Studies have shown fewer arrhythmias, heart attacks, and heart disease deaths in test subjects who previously had heart attacks while taking higher doses of omega-3s.

There is some evidence that omega-3 foods and supplements can check plaque build-up inside arteries and blood vessels thereby preventing strokes. Speak with your doctor if high levels of omega-3s might prove to be likely to produce a bleeding-related stroke due to health history.

The American Heart Association recommends two servings or more of fish per week. The fish with the highest omega-3s are the following: Anchovies, herring, lake trout, mackerel, salmon, and sardines. Choosing fish with a lower mercury content, such as catfish, pollock, tilapia, salmon, and shrimp is a very good strategy to keep in mind, particularly if it's being served to children. Limit albacore tuna to 6 ounces or less per week. Avoid smoked and salty fish, shark, swordfish, king mackerel and tilefish if you have high blood pressure. A serving is considered to be 3.5 ounces of cooked fish or ¾ cup of flaked fish.

It's been suggested by studies that depression, dementia, and age-related mental decline can be better managed by omega-3s. Studies continue to find a stronger connection, and no research touts fatty fish as a cure for any of these diagnoses. Check in with your doctor. No doubt these fatty acids will be prescribed as a part of an overall good health program that will assist in managing some related aging and mental health issues.

Other studies have found that omega-3s can suppress some of the symptoms of ADHD in children. Fatty fish in the diets of children diagnosed with attention deficit hyperactivity disorders does not replace treatment, but can support brain development and function.

Vegetarians have omega-3 options, too. Great sources of omega-3 are found in canola and flaxseed oil, broccoli, spinach, and edamame, commercially grown algae (wild algae may have unwanted toxins – better be safe), and walnuts.

Nightshade Vegetables

The vegetables in the nightshade category are a staple in many diets around the world. These vegetables are found in Mediterranean diets, among others. Some people get alarmed at the word "nightshade." If you have an auto-immune disease, you might do well to avoid these. Talk to your doctor first before consuming any. Nightshade vegetables also have a reputation with some people to aggravate arthritis pain. And some people may, indeed, seem to have increased joint pain from eating nightshade vegetables, but so far, there has been no scientific evidence to support that claim.

Nightshade plants have an intriguing, mysterious and "shady" history. Their questionable properties have been used to further plot in Shakespeare, Chaucer and in the Harry Potter series. Spooky stuff!

But, let's take a look at which ones have been cultivated for human consumption. These foods are anti-inflammatory and would fit into a diet geared toward supporting heart health, weight control, reducing arthritis pain, fighting against cancer, battling psoriasis, reducing LDL cholesterol, among a host of other amazing benefits. These nightshade vegetables are generally agreed to fight inflammation.

Tomatoes

Tomatoes have so many nutritious elements, they are considered a "Powerhouse" of nutrition. They've got potassium, iron, zinc and many other helpful compounds. They contain lycopene which is very beneficial in the reduction of pro-inflammatory compounds linked to several types of cancer. Lycopene is a carotenoid that is better digested with a fat-soluble substance. Cooking tomatoes in olive oil strengthens the body's ability to absorb lycopene. Tomatoes are also high in vitamin C, another compound that is a great anti-inflammatory substance.

Eggplant

This nightshade vegetable is found in many Mediterranean dishes. Think a little exotically. Recipes from Greece, Morocco, France and Turkey are considered Mediterranean foods, and lots of times eggplant will take a front row seat in a recipe from these countries. It tends to absorb the flavors of the various sauces within the recipes.

Why is it good for us? It improves heart and artery health, supports cognitive functioning and brain health, thanks to nasunin. Eggplants help with digestion and soothes stomach ulcers, cleans our blood, reduces risk of anemia, can be beneficial in treating insomnia. Eggplants have potassium, manganese, copper, vitamins B1, B3, and B6, folate, magnesium, tryptophan, and more. The anthocyanins protect heart health.

Such a humble fruit, although we think of it as a vegetable. Some even consider it as a berry. The smaller the eggplant, the better the taste. Steaming them rather than baking, boiling or frying them seems to preserve the anti-oxidants more fully.

Potatoes

Potatoes are a nightshade vegetable that have taken a bit of a rap currently, due to certain diets that limit the amount of carbohydrates to be consumed. But, take note of this. Their vitamin B assists with energy metabolism. Vitamin B breaks down carbohydrates converting them into glucose and amino acids, smaller compounds that create energy that's more accessible to the body. Potatoes have many healthful benefits that should be called to mind. We need to reframe our thinking about this versatile vegetable.

Potatoes contain iron, potassium, phosphorous, zinc and calcium and magnesium, and do much to maintain the strength and structure of bones. They provide vitamins B and C among lots of other minerals.

Iron supports many of the body's functions such as regulating body temperature, the gastrointestinal process, and the immune system. Approximately 10 million people in the United States are deficient in iron, and are at risk for anemia. A baked potato with the skin has more than 3 milligrams of iron, an important mineral that assists the protein, hemoglobin, to deliver oxygen to red blood cells.

The potassium, calcium, and magnesium found in white potatoes help to decrease blood pressure. The significant amounts of fiber provided by white potatoes lowers the amounts of cholesterol in the blood, thereby lessening the risk of heart disease.

Potatoes also contain folate, a B vitamin, that is regarded as an important factor in the prevention of cancer cells forming. Vitamin C reduces the severity and length of colds.

The fiber that white potatoes provide, helps fight against colorectal cancer.

There are so many benefits from white potatoes, but one more thing. An important nutrient called, choline, helps with early brain development as regards learning and memory. Pregnant women require choline for developing fetuses, along with the aforementioned iron.

Peppers

Bell peppers have a lot of tricks up their sleeves. They come in red, orange, yellow and green. The green bell peppers are unripe and are more bitter than the others. Peppers support night vision. They contain more than 200% of your daily vitamin C intake. Red bell peppers contain vitamin B and folate. They are low in calories and carbs and are comprised of 92% water, 2% fiber, and have a little protein and fat. They have wonderful anti-oxidant properties.

Spices

Three spices jump to mind that are nightshades. They are paprika, (dried and powdered red bell pepper), capsicum, and cayenne pepper. They all are capsaicinoids, which define them as anti-inflammatory. The capsaicinoid properties are what make them flare in your mouth. They are all considered nightshade vegetables. If they were sweet, such as a red, orange or yellow bell pepper, they'd be considered a fruit.

Capsicum is one of the most popular spices in Brazil and has anti-inflammatory properties. The nutritional profile of capsicum is impressive. It contains 404% of your daily need for vitamin C; 23% of your vitamin A; 15% of vitamin B6; 6% of your iron and magnesium each. Capsicum also contains potassium, protein, and dietary fiber. This spice seems to do it all:

1) It prevents damage to your hair follicles by encouraging blood flow to your scalp;

2) Skin care is made a little easier due to the anti-oxidants and phytochemicals that rejuvenate skin and help clear up rashes and eruptions;

3) It helps you feel full after a meal for longer, while it promotes digestion and reduces bloating and gas,

4) It combats cancer cells from forming,

5) The vitamin B and folate reduces levels of homocysteine that is linked to cardiovascular diseases. Capsicum reduces inflammation, improves joint health, builds immunity, and prevents iron deficiency (anemia). Flavonoids in capsicum defends against asthma, emphysema, and lung infections.

Paprika adds more than just a smoky flavor. Paprika reduces the signs of aging in our skin. The carotenoids that give paprika (and red bell peppers) their delightful color, go on the search for free-radicals that age our skin and the rest of our bodies. The use of paprika has been identified as a deterrent to developing rheumatoid arthritis. Paprika can protect our eye health with its rich wealth of lutein, zeaxanthin, vitamins A, as well as B6. The capsaicin, that which gives us the splash of burn, also inhibits cancer growth.

Cayenne pepper, that contains capsaicin, is a boon to those determined to lose weight and keep it off. It does this by changing the composition of gut bacteria, thereby reducing inflammation.

Studies have shown that those who consume chili peppers regularly have a 13% reduction of early mortality. Something to ponder.

Note About Deadly Nightshade Plants

Part of the concern that some people have with nightshade vegetables are that some nightshade plants contain the alkaloid called, solanine. Some have taxane. Others have coniine. These compounds can be dangerous in high concentrations. Just ask Socrates. These plants are referred to as "deadly nightshade." Here are a few of the most recognizable ones: Hemlock, being famous for the demise of Socrates. Daffodils' bulbs look surprisingly like edible onions. Just keep daffodils in the ground or in a vase. Oleander, a pink flower often found growing wild, is extremely toxic. Almost 100,000 suicides a year in Sri Lanka are purportedly due to the ingestion of this flower. Some of us have had the grim opportunity to use castor oil for constipation. Interestingly, castor beans are known to contain one of the most harmful substances on earth, ricin. None of our discussion has been centered around these "shady" plants for the very reasons you just now read about. We're not ever suggesting to add these to a salad. They have no place in your diet.

Inflammation is the result of lifestyle choices. Diet, lack of exercise, and stress results in the immune system releasing chemicals meant to battle injury and wounds, bacteria and viruses, even when there is no foreign invasion present.

Instead of having to go to the pharmacy, go to the grocery market or try a farmer's market. This will be the beginning of a set of practices that will feed your body, and give you energy and health. Eating these anti-oxidant foods, along with sleep, relaxation and exercise will reduce inflammation markers and will very likely curb your risk for illnesses.

Eggs

Eggs are among the most nutritious foods nature gave us. A whole egg contains almost every of the nutrients required to turn a single cell into a baby chicken.

A single large egg contains, among others:

- Vitamin A: 6% of the RDA

- Folate: 5% of the RDA

- Phosphorus: 9% of the RDA

- Selenium: 22% of the RDA

- Eggs also contain some amounts of vitamin D, vitamin E, vitamin K, vitamin B6, calcium and zinc needed by the human body on a daily basis

It is true that eggs are high in cholesterol, as a single egg contains almost 210 mg, which is over half of the recommended daily amount of 300 mg.

However, you should not forget that cholesterol does not necessarily raise cholesterol in the blood. This is because the liver produces large amounts of cholesterol every single day, but when you increase your intake amount of cholesterol, your liver simply produces less cholesterol.

However, people with genetic disorders like familial hypercholesterolemia might have to limit or avoid eggs.

On the top of this, eggs also raise HDL that stands for high-density lipoprotein, also known as the "good" cholesterol.

People who have higher levels of HDL usually have a lower risk of heart disease, stroke and other health problems

Eating eggs is a great way to increase HDL. In one study, eating two eggs per day for six weeks increased HDL levels by 10%.

Eggs also contain various trace nutrients that are very important for health.

Chapter 5: Lifestyle Changes – Exercise and Sleep

In ancient medicine, people were encouraged and expected to be active participants in their cures. The wise doctors of those times and cultures knew that if people had a strong belief in the methods being used and had a choice to be part of their wellness experience, the outcomes would be more positive, and even more reliable.

Western medicine is now taking a hard look back at these practices and the mind-set that is also focused toward preventative care. The new/old model is less passive and more interactive between what is prescribed by a doctor and that which is a patient's choice from various approaches toward health.

Yoga

More and more people, young and old, have chosen yoga as a way to strengthen their bodies, improve balance, calm the mind and relieve stress. This venerable practice of self-care has proven to be a legitimate way to achieve these goals, and provides a way for people to be involved in their care. It gives hope and empowerment to people to effect the changes they want to see in themselves.

There are many types yoga to choose from. A very popular style is *Hatha yoga*, a more physical type of yoga that concentrates on breath work, (*pranayama*), and incorporates poses (*asanas*). It is then followed by a rest period (*savasana*). Hatha is not so much a meditative yoga. But by focusing on breath, the mind seems to calm itself.

Hatha is actually any kind of yoga that focuses on postures that build strength and balance. Hatha is a rather general term to describe a style that is gentle and slow. The teaching can vary a lot. It's thought of as a great place for beginners to start.

There is a more fluid form, *Vinyasa*, that incorporates rapid movement into sun poses and breath work.

Power yoga and *Ashtanga* are more advanced types of yoga. Ashtanga is a fast-paced series of poses and always presented in the same order. Power yoga is a combination of both Vinyasa and Ashtanga and is an interpretation developed by Beryl Bender Birch and Bryan Kest which was designed to appeal to American students. Power yoga differs from Ashtanga in that there are no set series of poses. Instructors are free to mix up the poses. That makes it more accessible to individual classes and levels of ability.

Bikram yoga, with the same 26 copyrighted poses, will be used in any studio anywhere that offers Bikram. It incorporates 2 methods of breathing through the poses. This is what people are talking about when they say they are going to a "Hot Yoga" class. Students interested in flushing toxins out of their body are attracted to this style. The room is heated to 105 degrees Fahrenheit, and is kept at 40 percent humidity.

The repeated movements, chanting, stylized breathing techniques, and meditation are unique to *Kundalini yoga*. This practice, more advanced, focuses on moving energy from the base of the spine and out via the seven chakras, the points of spiritual power within the human body.

Although there are many more styles of yoga, *Restorative yoga* should be mentioned here for those new to yoga as a way to health and well-being. Restorative yoga offers a relaxing and gentle way to stretch and strengthen the body. The use of props such as blocks and bolsters assist with support as students move into poses that challenge balance.

Here is a quick list of benefits that have been more recently studied and affirmed by Western medicine:

- Improved muscle tone and strength
- Improved cardio health and circulation

- Lowers blood pressure
- Helps with attaining deeper sleep
- Detoxifies internal organs
- Increases flexibility and balance
- Releases endorphins that improve mood
- Helps decrease anxiety and depression
- Reduction in chronic pain

No doubt, any form of exercise from walking to lifting weights will improve strength and balance. But yoga is different. You won't find mirrors in yoga studios. One of the goals of yoga is to turn inward and to not bother with concerns that create anxiety. There is no worry about appearance or competing with other's ability. It's a time-proven way to achieve some of the nuances of health naturally.

Sleep

The older we get the more fragile sleep becomes. But even for children and young adults, sleep can be elusive. Due to worry, emotional factors, and physical discomfort getting a great night's sleep can be a challenge. It can even get to the point that just the thought of going to bed can create anxiety because of the dread of not being able to fall asleep or the inability to stay asleep.

People turn to pills hoping that that form of sleep aid will alleviate these problems. But holistic approaches to sleep are better for us. A more organic way to get to sleep will support and deepen sleep and promote natural sleep cycles that are often interrupted by waking consciousness.

Sleep hygiene has become almost a buzz word. But what does it mean? It's a practice that will defuse the mental inflammation that keeps us awake. We experience stress from junk light from phones and computers. We worry over finances, personal relationships and situations over which we have no control. Sleep hygiene is a way to prepare ourselves for the healing powers of sleep for our nervous system and for the rest of our bodies.

And why is sleep so important? Besides from being exhausted the next morning from not getting enough sleep or quality sleep, it can end up costing you your health. Here's why. Not enough sleep or even too much sleep can have the same effect on our immune system. Getting the right amount of sleep produces cytokines, the protein that protects our immune system fighting viruses and other foreign invaders. They also give your body the energy to heal itself from injury. If sleeping seems out of whack, cytokines aren't being produced the way they should be and your entire immune system can eventually be at risk for heart disease and diabetes.

What Isn't Sleep Hygiene

Just about everybody is undoubtedly a little guilty by indulging in these seemingly harmless behaviors before bed. But if they are part of a regular routine or are combined with two or three of these nighttime pre-sleep activities, it's no wonder so many of us are at least somewhat sleep deprived.

Using electronics - The blue light we get from sunlight provides us with energy and aids our attention so were more alert. However, contact with blue light emitted from Smartphones, televisions, computers and other digital devices are not what we need before bedtime. This blue light has short waves of light that penetrate all the way to the retina. Besides eye strain, this light reduces melatonin, the natural hormone that prepares you for sleep. There is even a body of thought that blue light from electronics may possibly be the causation of various cancers, diabetes, heart disease, and even obesity.

Alcohol, Caffeine and Cigarettes - Having a nightcap sounds soothing and sophisticated, but having alcohol too close to bedtime disrupts sleep. Over 27 studies have pointed out that imbibing inhibits rapid eye movement (REM) that part of the sleep cycle wherein we dream and is thought to be the most restorative. It's agreed that alcohol helps get people to sleep, but is disruptive in the second half of the sleep cycle spent trying to sleep whether it be night or day. Alcohol is also thought to precipitate sleep apnea symptoms because it suppresses breathing. Using alcohol as a sleep aid is risking memory problems, sleep walking and talking. Additionally, avoid caffeine and cigarettes because of their stimulant properties.

Vigorous Exercise – The jury is out on this. One school of thought is that exercise an hour or two before bedtime is fine. However, the other belief is that exercise should be finished with at least 4 hours ahead of bedtime. While exercising, your heart rate goes up and so does your core body temperature. Not conducive for sleeping. The hormones cortisol and adrenaline are stimulants which will keep some wide awake.

Figuring out what time to work out will be an individual thing. For some people struggling with sleep issues, a morning workout will be the answer. A study done by Appalachian State University found that people who pumped iron at 7 a.m. slept better than the group that lifted in the afternoons or at night or the people that didn't exercise at all. Yet those who worked out with weights at 7 p.m. slept the best. Confusing. Listen to your body.

Eating Before Bed – Nutritionists say eating a large meal 1 to 2 hours before bed isn't a good idea. It can disrupt sleep with possible heartburn. Weight gain is also a threat from eating a full meal so soon to bedtime. Both of these situations will only end up inflaming the immune system creating an environment for symptoms that can turn into chronic conditions.

Daytime Naps - It can be so tempting to lie down during the day, especially when one feels exhausted from lack of sleep the night before. But it often ends up making it almost impossible to get to sleep or sleep throughout the night. It creates a vicious cycle.

Good Sleep Hygiene

Set a regular sleep time in order to train your brain and body to "know" when it's time to get some rest. Take into consideration that life happens as they say, so if you're off 20 minutes early or late, you're still in a good sleep zone. If you have a habit of sneaking peeks at the clock, make sure you can't see its face.

Light Snacks – The experts are now saying that it's really more about what you eat rather than when you eat. It appears that it's okay to eat a small snack right before bed. Nutrient rich foods or a single macronutrient snack that will satiate hunger and feed your body while you sleep are good choices. These snacks would be a lean protein, a little fresh fruit, a small vegetable, a few walnuts, or a small serving of whole grain are permissible treats. The fitness gurus strongly suggest protein before bed if you have worked out that day. The sleep and protein fuel muscle repair.

Pre-Bedtime Routines - Establish a soothing pre-bedtime routine. This should be something you really look forward to in order to put a conclusion on your day. This could be a warm bath or shower to relax muscles and calm brain activity. Reading while sitting in a chair or sofa, not in bed, can now become a routine you never go without. Maybe meditate to calm the mind.

Environment - Create a space that will offer repose. The temperature should be a little cool, but comfortable. Get a comfortable bed, if you don't have one already. Some of the memory foam mattresses are reported to generate heat from your body that bounces back and forth between you and the mattress. This can disrupt sleep many times during the night. The room should be dark and pets that love to stretch out on the bed should be kept in another room. If a partner snores, then remedies to deal with that should be explored.

Set up an environment conducive to ASMR. ASMR, (autonomous sensory meridian response), is as old as time, but the attention and study of it is relatively new. It can be lots of things to lots of different people. Think of what we used to call "white sounds." It's typically a repetitive, monotonous but soothing sound. Some say it's sensuous. There are apps now that produce the sounds of the ocean, rain, sounds of brooks or rivers and many other sounds that relax and distract the mind letting you drift off to sleep. Getting your hair brushed or other massages are other examples of ASMR.

A good night's sleep helps our bodies to heal from injury or disease. Our brains work more efficiently and we suffer less from memory impairment if we have quality sleep. The deep sleep, the REM sleep, repairs and stimulates regions in the brain that are responsible for learning.

We have so many demands placed on us with our work, our family and our attempts to maintain a social support system. It's a temptation to forego sleep in order to get everything done. However, a pattern of quality sleep is crucial to our health. Take the time to develop habits that will ensure a good night's sleep.

Chapter 6: Anti-Inflammatory Supplements and Herbs

We have talked about how a quality diet keeps inflammation at bay. As you've been reading, so many environmental factors can bring on the unfortunate condition that degenerates our systems possibly establishing life-altering diseases. Inflammation has been called "The Silent Killer," because it's a major component of every disease from diabetes to Alzheimer's among others.

So, what else can you do to further reduce inflammation? The answer is really pretty simple. Aside from the recommended foods that control inflammation, adding vitamins, minerals, herbs and supplements to your diet can further reduce unwanted inflammation.

Vitamins

Before we get very far into this discussion about vitamins, it is recommended that you speak with your doctor about which vitamin supplements you should be taking. Talking about what form to take, what brand, prescribed or OTC, and what amount would be a conscientious thing to do. There can be negative results from medication interactions with additional consumption of vitamins. In the following pages, you will see some charts that offer basic guidelines to the amounts you would want to take. A conversation with your doctor and possibly a blood test might be in order before beginning a new regimen of vitamin supplements.

Taking vitamins A, B and C are an easy way to promote healing from inflammation. Recent research has found that these vitamins were inversely connected to prominent marker levels.

Vitamin A

Vitamin A is a fat-soluble vitamin that is great for skin, bones, vision as well as other tissues in the body. It has many other positive benefits aside from those.

Vitamin A is particularly helpful in the formation and maintenance of the heart, lungs and other vital organs.

One source for retinol, vitamin A, is based in animal products. It's referred to as pre-formed vitamin A. Most of these fats are not a part of an anti-inflammatory diet. However, feta and mozzarella are on the lower end of the saturated fat spectrum. Other hard cheeses are allowed as well.

Pro-vitamin A is plant based. This vitamin is found in brightly colored fruits and vegetables. Beta carotene, the pro-vitamin A found most often, can be found in cantaloupe, carrots, apricots, pumpkin, sweet potatoes, pink grapefruit. Beta-carotene is found in the dark, green leafy vegetables, too. Its antioxidant properties are responsible for fighting the free radicals that do damage to cells.

Vitamin A is beneficial in treating inflammation in acne and other skin conditions. It is essential for healthy eyes, especially with those who suffer dry eyes and cataracts. It's integral for general eye health, and particularly beneficial for night vision.

The popular Retin A products are regularly seen in skin care departments of department stores, pharmacies and over at the local grocery store. That's because it works by urging skin cells to grow at a faster rate, thereby making skin look fresh and youthful.

Vitamin B

Vitamin B is actually a conglomeration of 8 different vitamins. Some people can get all the vitamin B they need from their diet, but supplements are a good way to make sure you get a complete amount of this important vitamin.

The vitamin B complex ensures that your body can benefit from the energy it provides to cell growth. It assists in the healthy functioning of your internal organs, your nervous system, as well as your brain. It helps your body to process prescribed medicines. It addresses inflammation by breaking down fats into more manageable elements that are easier to digest. Vitamin B helps your body produce more red blood cells that defend against anemia.

Folate (B12)

Deficiencies in folate (vitamin B12) can establish an increased risk in many health issues such as: Alzheimer's disease, anemia, depression, heart disease, mouth ulcers, and nerve damage. Pregnant women low in folate face the risk of neural tube defects in their babies. Older people low in folate often feel short of breath and dizzy which can lead to falls.

Vitamin B12 deficiencies are rather common. This is a particular concern for people on a strict vegan diet, those taking long-term antacids for heartburn, people who have been prescribed Metformin for diabetes, those who have had a colon resection that removed the part of the bowel that absorbs B12, as well as the elderly.

There can be negative drug interactions with B12. Make sure to talk with your doctor about the appropriate amount you should be taking. Too much could create problems.

Vitamin C

Vitamin C has been proven being effective against the C-Reactive Protein. CRP is made by your liver in response to various threats to the body. If levels are chronically too high, the risk of multiple diseases from colds and flu to cancer can develop.

Of course, it is best to get the benefits from these vitamins, and others, through your diet, but there is the caveat that it can be impossible to attain all the requirements through food alone. If inflammation is a real concern, boosting the positive effects of vitamins and minerals through pill form is a boon. Finding quality sources for your vitamins is foremost.

Minerals

Copper

Copper aids in the early recovery and healing from injury and surgery. It reduces production of free radicals that damage cells and develop cancer. Copper also limits the number of white blood cells. We know a proliferation of white blood cells set us up for infection. Not having enough copper in your system can allow for the development of osteoporosis. This condition weakens bones and makes them more at risk for breakage. Copper aids in collagen production that helps skin stay looking youthful. Our brain functioning is supported by appropriate copper levels.

Iron

When you haven't been pumping your "iron," so to speak, you may feel weak and fatigued, possibly have some chest pain and a fast heartbeat. Maybe people have teased you saying that you have "cold hands but a warm heart." Maybe you feel dizzy and light-headed, and crave non-nutritive foods. All joking aside, you may be iron deficient. But don't diagnose yourself! Do see a doctor about these signs.

Iron deficiency happens when your blood doesn't have enough iron to produce hemoglobin. Hemoglobin is the part of red blood cells that make blood look red and make them capable of carrying oxygen to all parts of your body.

Sometimes your diet can cause you to become iron deficient. If you aren't eating enough lean meat, eggs and dark green, leafy vegetables that might be the cause.

Women who have heavy periods can become iron deficient. Other causes of blood loss such as a colon polyp, hiatal hernia, undetected colon cancer, peptic ulcers can cause this deficiency. Continual use of aspirin or other over the counter pain relievers can cause gastrointestinal bleeding.

Celiac disease can lead to anemia because of the intestines inability to digest and absorb nutrients from your food. Pregnant women can sometimes be at risk because their hemoglobin needs to provide for their growing fetus as well as themselves.

Zinc

A zinc deficiency can possibly be indicated by a decreased of smell and taste, and could be linked to a loss of appetite. Other indicators include unexplained weight loss, unexplained sores on the skin and wounds that won't heal. It's responsible for lack of alertness and even hair loss.

Zinc's job is to produce new cells and to fight off infections. It's needed to maintain cell and DNA health. It's necessary for sexual development. A deficiency can be linked to impotency in men. Zinc deficiency is rare in the U.S., but it still occasionally develops in people.

Vegans and vegetarians can be at risk for developing this deficiency. Consider adding more almonds, baked beans, peas and cashews to your diet. To ward off a lack of zinc for meat eaters, be sure to include red meat and poultry, whole grains and even oysters.

Zinc deficiency can be diagnosed through a hair sample, or a urine or blood test.

Herbs

Ancient medical practitioners have long used herbs and spices to treat a wide variety of physical ailments. The use of these "medicines" was thought to be extremely powerful based on their understanding of the anti-inflammatory and anti-oxidant properties contained within herbs and spices. And they were right.

Although not using these same medical terms, the ancient physicians knew that inflammation and oxidation are closely related. Anti-oxidants stop the development of inflammation of cells from the destruction done by free radicals. Good nutrition can ward off inflammation by switching off genes that establish inflammatory processes. These nutrients alter the gut biome and concentrate the proteins that fight inflammation. Adding herbs and spices to your diet can invigorate the way your diet protects you from inflammatory diseases.

This essential ability is highly concentrated in spices and herbs. For example, a half teaspoon of dried oregano has as many anti-oxidants as three cups of spinach. A half teaspoon of cinnamon has as many anti-oxidants as a half cup of blueberries. Impressive!

Spices are an easy way to boost our body's defense against inflammation. It's easy to sprinkle these fighters into many dishes and make yourself look like a master chef at the same time! Here are some that you probably already have in your spice rack at this very moment.

Turmeric

Turmeric is considered the strongest anti-inflammatory her. The herb turmeric has an anti-oxidant compound called curcumin. Curcumin gives curry and mustard that golden color, which are good food sources for this anti-oxidant. Many people report that taking turmeric soothes the effects of arthritis. One study has shown that it relieves pain as well or better than ibuprofen.

Turmeric can protect your liver from being damaged by toxins. People being treated aggressively for cancer or diabetes often are prescribed turmeric supplements to boost the function of their livers.

Both Ayurvedic and Chinese medicine utilized turmeric to address patients' ills from arthritis to liver disease, immune disorders and dementia. These physicians were very wise.

Green Tea

"It's the healthiest thing I can think of to drink," raves Christopher Ochner, PhD, a research scientist from the Ichan School of Medicine at Mt. Sinai Hospital. It's a particularly healthful drink because of the catechin content. Green tea is processed very little so the level of anti-oxidants in the catechin is high. Catechins are linked to preventing cancer. Green tea drinkers are less likely to experience prostate and breast cancer. More studies are suggesting that green tea lowers chances of developing type 2 diabetes.

Green tea has been shown to boost metabolism and increases fat burning. Other studies indicate that green tea promotes burning additional calories every day. Other possible benefits from consuming green tea are improved dental health, and improved brain function. MRI's from a Swiss study showed that the working memory areas in the brains of test subjects had greater activity. It has been linked to a lower risk of Parkinson's and Alzheimer's diseases.

Green tea has been credited with reducing blood pressure, and lowering cholesterol. Green tea has been credited in reducing oral cancer in an observational study of women who drank three to four cups of this tea per day. In a larger observational study, green tea consumption was linked a reduced risk of stomach cancer in women who drank 5 or more cups per day.

Other studies have shown a reduction in prostate cancer, pancreatic cancer and breast cancer.

The green tea that is hand-picked is thought to be milder and sweeter than the tea that's harvested by machine. Green tea is grown in higher altitudes than black tea. Black tea ferments which alters its color and flavor. Green tea isn't processed the way black tea is, and so retains its flavor and color.

There are several types of green tea. Two of the most popular are Matcha and Sencha. All green teas have a high chlorophyll content, which makes for the bright green color in the leaf. When Matcha is processed, the leaf is ground to a powder, and mixed with boiling water to produce a sweet flavor.

Sencha, is a popular green tea in Japan. Sencha leaves are steamed and then shaped. It produces a light green-yellow tea with a grassy and astringent flavor.

Cinnamon

The herb, cinnamon, has been recorded since 2,800 BC as an essential kitchen spice. But recently, many trial studies are exploring its benefits in treating Parkinson's disease, lowering blood pressure, calming inflammation in the brain, defeating cancer and managing diabetes.

Many patients long-treated for diabetes come to the point where the medicines are no longer effective. There have been several small trials that have seen some evidence that cinnamon helps regulate blood glucose levels. Ten controlled trials with over 500 patients wherein doses of cinnamon taken in doses of 120 mg to 6 g per day for a period of 4 months were linked to a decrease in levels of fasting plasma glucose along with a correction in lipid panels.

The phytochemicals found in cinnamon supports the brain in processing glucose. This has been witnessed in studies by the decrease in the number of markers in oxidative stress in rats. Cinnamon has an been found to support insulin resistance, thereby reducing Alzheimer's alterations in the brain.

Rosemary

For centuries, rosemary has been used in cooking and in folk medicine. It is an evergreen shrub and a member of the mint family. It is related to lavender, oregano and thyme. It has been renowned for its role in the culinary world, but it has also had a large presence as a medicinal compound. Rosemary has been traditionally used to minimize muscle pain, improve concentration, assist in digestion and to prevent baldness.

For thousands of years, rosemary was often used to treat pain. Nowadays, rosemary has been studied to determine how true those claims are. In a two-week study, rosemary was identified as an effective pain reliever for stroke survivors with shoulder pain. They were given a rosemary oil blend in conjunction with acupuncture for 20 minutes twice a day and experienced a 30% reduction in pain. Those who received only the acupuncture experienced only a 15% amount of pain reduction.

Inhaling rosemary oil may reduce stress. A study was done with nursing students that breathed rosemary oil from an inhaler before and during their tests. It was determined that their pulse decreased by about 9 percent. It was reported that no significant change in pulse rate was experienced by those who did not not breathe the essential oil. Another small study found that when young adults inhaled rosemary oil for 5 minutes, their saliva had 23% less cortisol as opposed to the group who inhaled only a placebo.

Rosemary improves circulation. Thermal imaging has confirmed that when rosemary oil is rubbed into the hands there is evidence that warmth is produced. Rosemary may be assisting by expanding blood vessels thereby moving blood to extremities. Interesting prospects, but further study needs to be completed to confirm related findings.

Oil of rosemary has been identified to promote hair growth. In a comparative study done in 2015, rosemary was found to be more effective than minoxidil 2% at treating androgenic alopecia cases by supporting hair growth. It increases microcirculation of the scalp and reduces hair loss after shampooing.

Rosemary is a good source of vitamin B-6, iron, and calcium. The effective compound, rosmarinic acid, has been identified to be an anti-inflammatory and an anti-oxidant. In 2003, a study published in the *Journal of Rheumatology* stated that this effective compound, rosmarinic acid, slowed the development of rheumatoid arthritis in laboratory mice.

Rosemary oil may help reduce tissue inflammation that leads to pain, swelling and stiffness according to preliminary studies. In a two-week trial, people with rheumatoid arthritis were given 15-minute knee massages three times a week with a rosemary oil application. At the end of the study, it was reported that those receiving this treatment had a 50% decrease of inflammatory pain. Those that received massages without the rosemary oil were reported to only having a 15% decrease in pain.

Rosemary suppresses beta amyloid plaque which is a primary cause in the development of dementia and Alzheimer's disease as was shown in a study published by Dr. Solomon Habtemariam. The research was entitled: "Brain Food for Alzheimer-Free Ageing: Focus on Herbal Medicines." The study also associated rosemary with stimulating cognitive activity in those suffering from acute cognitive disorders and declining cognitive activity in the elderly.

A 2016 study identified that the carnosic acid in rosemary is effective in reducing overstimulation in nerve cells and impacts oxidative stress thereby ultimately protecting the nervous system. It's also been shown to protect certain parts of the brain from damage done by ischemic injury.

The journal *Nutrition and Cancer* published a 2015 report that linked rosemary extract to the treatment of cancer. Rosemary extracts have anti-inflammatory properties as well as antiproliferative, antioxidant and anticancer properties that selectively kill cancer cells. Promising results have been identified in the treatment of pancreatic cancer, colon cancer, breast, bladder, cervical, ovarian and prostate cancers.

Clove

During the 13th and 14th centuries, merchants transported cloves all the way from Indonesia to India, China, Persia, Europe and Africa. Wars were fought over the production and distribution of this costly spice. The island of Maluku saw battles for control of clove production during both Medieval times and more recent times. The Dutch controlled the islands of Maluku and the clove industry for many years.

For thousands of years, the Chinese and Indians used the spice as a condiment and as a medicine to treat many illnesses. Ayurvedic medicine applied cloves to treat halitosis and tooth decay. The Chinese believed clove to be an aphrodisiac. Chinese courtiers of the court placed cloves in their mouths to ensure that their breath smelled fresh before having audience with the Emperor.

The USA National Nutrient Database has identified the following nutrients found in cloves. Cloves contain calcium, potassium, magnesium and sodium. Vitamins that were identified as components in clove are A, K, C, and E, as well as folate and niacin. They contain iron, phosphorous and zinc. They are little powerhouses full of anti-inflammatory properties.

Cloves stimulate the production of digestive enzymes and have been found useful in the treatment of flatulence, dyspepsia, gastric irritability and nausea. They have been roasted, powdered and mixed with honey for treatment of digestive disorders. It's been used as a remedy for dysentery and chronic diarrhea.

A study published by the *Oxford Journal: Carcinogenesis* identified clove as being helpful in controlling early cell growth in lung cancer. Research has linked the oleanolic acid found in cloves to antitumor activity and has anticancer properties against cervical cancer.

The phenolic compounds such as eugenol found in cloves have been identified as being helpful in preserving bone density. It assists in protecting the mineral content of bone in addition to adding tensile strength of bones in people diagnosed with osteoporosis.

The compound eugenol is what gives cloves the power to fight inflammation in heart disease and cancer. There has been a number of studies on eugenol particularly as it relates to the prevention of toxicity from environmental pollutants and is proving to be effective.

In animal studies eugenol has been added to diets that are high in anti-inflammatory foods. Some research has shown that the addition of eugenol has further reduced inflammation by as much as 30%. One test-tube study showed that eugenol arrested oxidative damage caused by free radicals five times more successfully than vitamin E.

The essential oil of clove is also popular in aromatherapy. Its scent stimulates the brain making you feel more attentive and energetic.

Ginger

Ginger is a popular culinary spice that has powerful medicinal properties. It contains gingerol and shogaol, anti-inflammatory agents that have been shown to offer many advantages to aid in our health. It aids in digestion. It reduces heartburn and acid reflux. One study found that taking 1,200 mg of ginger with a meal hastens digestion and the gastric emptying process by double. You'll then be able to absorb more quickly the vitamins and anti-inflammation properties from the food you eat. When food sits in the gut waiting to be digested, it saps energy from us.

Many other anti-inflammatory benefits are derived from ginger. It assists in the treatment of hypertension which affects your arteries, your heart, your brain, your kidney and even eyes.

Ginger has anti-bacterial properties that aid in warding off e-coli and reduce the pathogens that produce periodontitis. It lowers cholesterol levels and is a power blood sugar regulator.

Hypertension is a common result of processed foods that are so prevalent in the typical American diet. When hypertension is left untreated, it can do irreparable damage to your brain, your heart, your arteries, kidneys and eyes. Ginger, acts as a vasodilator, expanding blood vessels. It helps to reduce blood pressure by increasing circulation in the body. Ginger also contains potassium, also assisting in the treatment of high blood pressure.

Ginger has been identified as an anti-nausea remedy for nausea associated with chemotherapy and pregnancy. It's been found to reduce the nausea related to seasickness. Additionally, ginger has been identified by researchers to be "an effective means for reducing post-operative nausea and vomiting."

Researchers have identified ginger as an effective anti-bacterial for several drug-resistant bacteria in clinical settings. In that study researchers said: "Ginger has great potential in the treatment of many microbial diseases (such as Bacillus and E. coli)."

Ginger is effective in managing cholesterol levels. According to the American Heart Association, "LDL cholesterol is called 'bad' cholesterol. Think of it as less desirable or even lousy cholesterol, because it contributes to fatty build ups in arteries." Atherosclerosis is the name of this fatty build up, which increases the risk of heart attack and stroke. Using ginger in your cooking is a way to inhibit the growth of fatty build up.

Ginger is a versatile herb. It can be found in teas. People are finding that ginger milk is a soothing bedtime drink. Ginger spritzers are popular. It can be added to smoothies. Ginger water has become a thing. There are now many recipes for main dishes and sides that require this anti-inflammatory spice.

Fennel

Apart from being used in the kitchen for thousands of years, fennel has benefits that are beyond the culinary realm. It has a unique combination of phytonutrients such as rutin, quercetin, anethole and kaempferol glycosides which make this seed a powerful antioxidant.

Of these phytonutrients, anethole has been shown to be the most effective in reducing inflammation and preventing cancer.

Fennel contains vitamin C, the body's primary water-soluble antioxidant that neutralizes free radicals that create inflammation in all areas of the body. Free radicals have been proven to cause cellular damage resulting in joint deterioration and pain that occurs in osteo and rheumatoid arthritis.

Fiber removes potentially carcinogenic toxins from the colon. Fennel is a great source of fiber. It's been suggested that fennel is a way to boost the fight against colon cancer.

In addition, fennel has the element of potassium. The mineral potassium is important in the reduction of high blood pressure which is a risk factor in stroke and heart attacks.

Fennel has also been found to suppress appetite by instilling a feeling of being full and satisfied. It boosts metabolism while breaking down fats into the blood stream into more useable and digestible elements of nutrition. In a study done in 2006, *The Journal of Animal Physiology and Animal Nutrition* published findings that fennel was found to be helpful in regulating over eating.

This herb has been long considered to be an important natural diuretic aiding in the formation and secretion of urine, thereby decreasing water retention. Fennel has been credited in preventing osteoporosis. It contains multiple nutrients including calcium, iron, phosphorus, magnesium, manganese, vitamin K and zinc that help to build bones and maintain their strength. A study published in the *International Journal of Molecular Medicine* in 2002, reported that eating fennel seeds improved bone mineral density and content in post-menopausal women suffering from post-menopausal bone loss and osteoporosis.

Garlic

Garlic, an anti-inflammatory herb, has an intriguing and fun history! King Tut's tomb was found to be littered with bulbs of garlic. Fifteen pounds of garlic, in Egyptian times, would have purchased a male slave. It was considered a "performance enhancement" tool by Greeks. Roman generals had their soldiers plant garlic in the fields of conquered countries so that the bulb would provide strength and courage to their troops when eaten. Ancient Indian lore regarded garlic as an aphrodisiac. In the Middle Ages, garlic was worn around the neck to ward off werewolves. Later, people wore garlic to defend themselves against contagious diseases.

Garlic is a cousin of the onion, as well as the lily. It is added to many dishes found in many different cultures. This anti-oxidant offers protection against many diseases. This herb has been used to prevent lung and prostate cancers, breast, stomach, renal and colon cancer, as well. Studies found in peer-reviewed academic articles have relayed the following information: People that ate garlic twice a week, over a 7-year study, experienced 44% lower risk of developing lung cancer. The compound organosulfur, found in garlic, has been identified by the Medical University of South Carolina to be a strong deterrent to the development of brain cancer cells. Kings College in London supports the findings that garlic, shallots, leeks and onions can lower levels of osteoarthritis in women used as test subjects. The *Journal of Antimicrobial Chemotherapy* found that diallyl sulfide, a compound in garlic, was found to be 100 times more effective than two widely-used antibiotics.

Garlic has been used as a treatment for heart failure. Garlic, with its anti-oxidant properties reduces diastolic and systolic blood pressures. It has been studied and seen that it lowers cholesterol and lowers blood pressure.

Allium vegetables (onions, leeks, shallots), but particularly garlic, have been studied to see if there is a connection between consumption and the reduction of prostate cancer. The *Asian Pacific Journal of Cancer Prevention* in May 2013 revealed the findings that garlic is related to reduction of prostate cancer.

From reducing the incidence of pre-term labor to the reduced frequency of the common cold, garlic is an important anti-inflammatory herb to include in our diets.

Sage

Thousands of years ago, sage was used as an antidote to snakebite. It was also used by ancient Egyptians to boost fertility in females. Sage has been used in the past for spiritual cleansing. Burning sage in a new home was thought to be a way to rid the home of bad energy. It is still done by many. Now, most people associate sage with the fragrance of the holidays. When we walk into the door at mom's on Thanksgiving or Christmas morning, the smell of sage from the turkey or dressing is one of the things that really brings us back home.

Sage has been widely used in Chinese Ayurvedic medicine. Traditional herbalists have used sage to treat a variety of ailments and sicknesses that include pain relief, infection, bleeding gums and sore throat, even ulcers. Herbalists would prepare sage tea to ease the pain of severe menstrual cramps, aid digestion and address diarrhea.

Currently, sage is being researched for its many possible uses in the treatment of a wide array of disorders. Researchers at the Department of Pharmacology and Toxicology at the University of Otago in New Zealand are taking a serious look at the way Spanish sage works against Alzheimer's disease in both rats and humans. Test subjects experienced lessening of neuropsychiatric symptoms and a boost in mental attention. Sage was, therefore, credited for its ability to help mental capabilities in patients with dementia and Alzheimer's.

Researchers at the Northumbria University in England reported that there was a clear, general improvement in the "alertness," "calmness," and "contentedness" in patient's strong negative emotions and agitation who are dealing with the terrible experience of Alzheimer's and dementia.

In animal studies, sage has been proven to lower glucose levels. Research scientists at the University of Minho in Portugal gave both mice and rats a sage tea to evaluate its antidiabetic effects. They found that its "metformin-like effects on rat hepatocytes suggest that sage may be useful as a food supplement in the prevention of type 2 diabetes mellitus by lowering the plasma glucose of individuals at risk."

Additionally, the mice that were fed a high-fat diet to promote obesity were treated with sage in order to find benefits of sage in treating diabetes. These mice were treated for five weeks with either a control substance or with sage methanol extract. The results were that the mice that were treated with the sage methanol extract were reported to have insulin sensitivity improvements, as well as a reduction in inflammation. It was concluded that "sage presents an alternative to pharmaceuticals for the treatment of diabetes and associated inflammation."

The Journal of Molecular Sciences published findings about a pilot study that evaluated the benefits of sage tea on women, aged 40 to 55, on blood glucose regulation, reduction in cholesterol and lipid profiles. It was revealed that after 4 weeks of sage tea there was "an improvement in lipid profile was observed with lower plasma LDL cholesterol and total cholesterol levels as well as higher plasma HDL levels during and after two weeks after treatment."

It is well known that obesity is known to be the primary contributor to type 2 diabetes, hypertension and a collection of other health issues. Weight loss products seem to flood the shelves of pharmacies and grocery stores. It's been found by numerous studies that the methanolic extract from sage leaves counters the absorption of fat in the pancreas. Also found was the overall body weight loss in mice that were fed a high-fat diet and were given the same methanolic extract.

The salvia species have been utilized in the treatment of depression, memory disorders and cerebral ischemia. It has been used for centuries to restore declining mental functions. Sage is now being studied for its protection against Alzheimer's and other inflammation-based neurological conditions such as epilepsy, Parkinson's disease and stroke. The mood enhancing properties are being considered as an application in the treatment of agitation in dementia patients. A recent study has shown that sage improves cognition and the speed of recovering memory.

It boosts the immune system, regulates digestion, strengthens bones, improves skin conditions, and prevents diabetes. The herb has been researched for its ability to support concentration and restore memory. It has been suggested that increased brain activity after ingesting sage positively impacts focus and memory. However, further study will clarify how true that is.

In analyzing just one tablespoon of sage, the following nutrients have been identified: 34.3 micrograms of vitamin K, 33 milligrams of calcium, 118 international units of vitamin A, and 8.6 milligrams of magnesium. There are also trace amounts of protein, fat, fiber, vitamin B, iron and manganese. Sage offers huge anti-inflammatory benefits. But it's wise to keep in mind that other herbs, spices and foods must be included to round out an anti-inflammatory diet.

Frankincense

Frankincense is a resin extracted from Boswellia trees. These trees are native to Ethiopia, India, Somalia and the Arabian Peninsula. This resin is currently being used to treat inflammatory and degenerative joint disorders.

Boswellia and curcumin together have been found even more efficient at treating osteoarthritis than a popular synthetically made drug.

Frankincense in an essential oil form is used by many rheumatoid arthritis sufferers for pain relief. Frankincense isn't used to treat the disease of RA, but is very often a mainstay in the pain management. It has been shown in various studies to reduce inflammation, pain and stiffness. Frankincense, in laboratory settings, to have positive immune system effects.

Maritime Bark (Pycnogenol)

This herb is an extremely effective extract to reduce vascular inflammation, heal wounds and treat ulcers. It is identified as one of the strongest anti-inflammatory herbs. Studies have confirmed that pycnogenol is 50-100 times stronger than vitamin E in neutralizing free radicals. It lessens the risk of blood clots and reduces blood pressure.

It is used to treat allergies, asthma, high blood pressure, osteoarthritis, diabetes, endometriosis, attention deficit hyper-activity disorder (ADHD), and retinopathy, a disease of the eye.

Pcynogenol is used to relieve symptoms that postmenopausal women experience. That conclusion was drawn based on the anti-oxidative effects on the endothelium, the thin membrane found inside blood vessels and within the heart. In this same study, it was shown that pycnogenol boosts nitric oxide availability assisting in circulation.

Another study found that pcynogenol is linked to reducing the pain and swelling in chronic venous insufficiency, when veins have difficulty returning blood from the legs back to the heart.

A 2009 research study involving people in the early stages of diabetes and diabetic retinopathy showed that 18 of the 24 participants had improved vision. Those who took the placebo experienced no change in their vision.

It's an anti-inflammatory used in preventing heart disease and stroke. It reduces the occurrence of varicose veins and is found in many "anti-aging" products. Maritime bark capsules can be found online or at your nearest health product store.

Chapter 7: The Lifestyle Approach

We want to get to a place where we can enjoy our new health and the way our bodies and minds feel from eliminating the toxins we have been consuming with poor diet choices for so long. To complete this new life experience, there are practices that will enhance your new quality of life. Let's take a look at some of them.

Clicking Off Technology

Especially in this day and age, we are surrounded by technology that was first intended to bring people together. We were told that with an email, a quick text, a phone call, or video that this would create a way to reach out, create, inform and help build relationships. Funny thing is, it seems to work the other way for lots of us.

There is a general feeling in our world of a lack of permanence and a lot of emptiness. How can we recreate a fuller life and sustain that? Here are some thoughts and suggestions on getting ourselves back to a place where we feel present, calm, clear-thinking and available to ourselves and others.

Research is saying that many of us touch our screens 2,617 times a day. That seems like a lot. But even if we aren't one of those people, and let's hope we're not, you know that most of us are pretty phone-obsessed. We are constantly interrupted by others sending us information and by ourselves checking texts, emails, the weather, the news, ordering food, making purchases, finding directions, playing games and more. We're available to others 24/7 which is very stressful.

It's been proven that technology, especially Smartphones, is addicting. There is a surge of endorphins every time we open a text, email, some kind of social media site or even by checking the air quality on our phones. Endorphins are the hormone that gives us the "Feel Goods." It works just like alcohol, just like marijuana or other substances that alter our moods.

Blue light exposure from screens puts people at risk for what is being called "Computer Face." That face has premature wrinkles, frown lines, jowls, furrowed foreheads and 'turkey neck.' Another name for it is 'screen dermatitis.' Screen time also contributes to eye strain.

Social media sites like Facebook are contributing to what researchers call "Fear of Missing Out" (FOMO for short). Social media streams all the wonderful activities, amazing vacations, birthday greetings, and gatherings with friends and family that not everyone has access to. People end up feeling left out and even inadequate. Girls and young women are particularly vulnerable to FOMO. It sets up a mental environment ripe for loneliness and depression no matter what age or gender you are.

Of course, not everything about technology is bad. It's the way we use it that gets in our way to a fuller life.

So, what to do?

First of all, we need to embrace the idea that real life is right in front of us. There are moments and experiences that will never be repeated. The sunrise or sunset of this day will never happen again. If we're glued to technology, we'll miss those conversations with people we care about. Our kids and our pets and our significant others may not be around when we turn away from our screens and think we're ready to interact. This should be our motivation when we think about cutting back on technology.

Let's start with phones. Make meal times a "Phone Free Time." This will help us connect to others and to ourselves. It was once thought rude for people to take calls during meal times. That seems to have loosened up a lot with the more prevalent use of phones. And guess what. It's still rude. Granted there are people with professions who do have to be available 24 hours a day, at least on scheduled days. That doesn't apply here. The rest of the time, phones should be turned off when the meal isn't being served. Even turning off notifications but leaving it sitting in front of us is still a temptation for lots of us. Put it away.

Schedule "coffee breaks" from your phone. Give yourself even 15 minutes a couple of times a day to take a break. But don't rely on just yourself to discipline yourself to do this. It sounds ironic, but set your phone to alert you of your break times. Then leave it somewhere where it will be unavailable for that time.

If you are one of those who check their phones at traffic lights, put the phone in the backseat or even the trunk if you have to. Play music instead. Talk to your passenger, if you have one. Your passenger will thank you and so will all the other drivers on the road whether you can hear them or not. Getting directions from our phones is pretty standard these days. If possible, give a passenger the phone to tell you what turn to take next.

Inform people about your new boundaries. Let them know when it's okay for them to try to contact you or when it's likely that you'll be able to get back to them. If you don't, you'll end up having to apologize. You'll end up having to get back to your screen and then lose control of your free time.

Screen time has a strong connection to consumerism. You'll probably find that by being mindful of your screen time, you're spending a whole lot less money on things that you don't really need. Instead, take that money and put it to use to enjoy experiences with people you care about. Or maybe spend some money and time on a getaway for yourself to relax and heal from life's demands. It doesn't need to be extravagant.

Walking

In chapter 5, we talked about yoga as an approach to strengthen your body, to improve energy and vitality and achieve some peace and tranquility in this hectic world.

Another form of exercise that will provide social, emotional and physical strength is walking. Walking supports many aspects of a healthy lifestyle. Walking is easier on the joints and heart than running or jogging. Walking is now being hailed as "the closest thing we have to a wonder drug" according to former director of Centers for Disease Control and Prevention, Dr. Thomas Frieden. Many positive gains from this form of exercise are available to most. Even starting out with a small walk can evolve into much looked forward to regimen. Let's look at some of the things walking can do for you.

Oxygen and Circulation

As you walk, the improved circulation supplies the brain with the required oxygen and glucose for optimum functioning. You can even become a little smarter by walking! By bringing up the heart rate and lowering blood pressure, you are protecting both your heart and brain. University of Colorado at Boulder and the University of Tennessee found in their studies that post-menopausal women were able to lower their blood pressure by 11 points in 6 months. Thirty minutes of walking a day were linked to a 20 percent less risk of stroke in a similar study group, and by stepping up the pace, risk of stroke was reduced by 40 percent.

Staying Hydrated

The human body is 60 percent water. Staying hydrated after exercise and through-out the day only makes sense to maintain maximum function of our brains, the heart, the transportation of nutrients to cells and to flush out toxins.

Weight Loss - Staying hydrated assists with weight loss. The results of several studies reported in the journal *Obesity* showed that more weight was lost by those who regularly drank the recommended amount of water than those who did not.

Cardiovascular Health - Drinking water lowers the risk of heart attacks. When dehydrated, arteries become narrow. If there is cholesterol and plaque being stored within these arteries, the risk of heart attacks becomes very high. Keeping hydrated improves the way arteries function.

Flushing Toxins - The elimination of waste is hindered by being dehydrated. The kidneys and colon rely on being hydrated in order to function properly. Being hydrated prevents the occurrence of kidney stones. Proper hydration protects against rheumatoid arthritis and eases the pain of osteoarthritis.

Boosts Energy Levels - The *Journal of Athletic Training and Nutrition* published findings that staying hydrated before, during and after exercising not only lessened fatigue, but also boosted endurance.

Avoid the single-use plastic water bottles. Besides polluting the environment with discarded plastic, drinking out of these bottles isn't good for us. Plastic bottles contain bisphenol A (BPA), a chemical used to make the plastic clear and durable. It's an endocrine disruptor and has been linked to neurological issues, cancer, and early puberty in young girls among other problems. BPA has been found in growing fetuses and placentas.

Also found in the plastic of water bottles and other food storage containers is another chemical called phthalates, which is another endocrine disruptor. Presently, the FDA doesn't regulate phthalates as it is found in trace amounts in plastic. But when you consider the frequency that plastic is used as a container, it really is prevalent in our lives.

Utilize metal water bottles to keep the hydration process safe. They can be washed again and again. The purity of the water from plastic has been debated over the past few years. It's typically only as clean as tap water.

Be good to yourself. Stay hydrated. Choose a method that will match an anti-inflammatory lifestyle.

Walking Boosts Immunity

Walking counteracts the effects of weight-producing genetics. Researchers at Harvard examined 32 weight producing genes to evaluate how they contribute to body weight. Over 12,000 people were part of the study. It was discovered that those who walked briskly every day for an hour the effect of these genes was cut by 50 percent.

Researchers agree that any sort of exercise helps prevent certain types of cancer. Walking actually prevents the formation of breast cancer. The American Cancer Society conducted a study of women who walked at least 7 hours per week. It was discovered that these women had a 14% reduced risk of developing breast cancer compared to women who only walked 3-4 hours per week.

Just by walking 30 minutes a day, your immune cells are strengthened with oxygen improving the function of B-cells, T-cells and releases clumps of WBCs (white blood cells) found in the renal system and urinary tract. A study of 1,000 men and women reported that during the cold and flu season walkers had a 43 percent lower chance of getting sick. By walking only 20 minutes a day for at least 5 days a week, the test group experienced fewer symptoms and a shorter duration of colds and flu, if they became sick at all.

Walking Strengthens Bones

The gentle strike of your feet against the sidewalk, ground or track squeezes the cartilage sending oxygen and nutrients to your joints. Walking produces vitamin D, which nourishes bones. You'll experience a reduction in joint pain because of this nutritious lubrication and makes the threat of osteoarthritis less likely. This is really important to arthritis sufferers. Muscles around the joints are strengthened. Studies have shown that 5 miles a week can ward off the development of arthritis in the first place.

Slows Mental Decline

A study of 6,000 women, age 65 plus at the University of California, San Francisco found that there was a significant decline in age-related memory issues. From walking 2.5 miles per day, there was a 17 percent decline in memory as opposed to those women who only walked a half mile per day. The second group suffered declines at 25 percent.

Walking reduces the risk of Alzheimer's. The group of men ages of 71 to 93 studied at the University of Virginia Health System in Charlottesville, had half the incidence of Alzheimer's disease if they walked more than a quarter of a mile a day than those men who walked less.

If you walk regularly at a moderate pace, a pace wherein you can still hold a conversation, your risk of Alzheimer's and impaired memory is largely decreased.

Longer Lives

People who regularly exercise by walking in their fifties and sixties are 35 percent more likely to live longer than those who do not walk. A Harvard study of 17,000 graduates showed that they lived longer than their sedentary peers. A study by the American Geriatrics Society determined that people between the ages of 70 to 90 who maintained some sort of physical activity lived longer than their counterparts.

It appears that all forms of inflammatory diseases can improve with regular walking. A more recent study from *Arthritis and Therapy* suggested that interval walking improves the immune function in people with rheumatoid arthritis. David Nieman, professor of public health at Appalachian State University, as well as being the director of the Human Performance Lab there, has spent nine years studying the effects of exercise on the immune system. He said, "We found that, after three hours of exercise, these immune cells retreat back to the tissues they came from." This means that when immune cells come across destructive pathogens, they are able to destroy them.

You may have heard of Blue Zones. These are parts of the world where people live longer than the average. The term *"Blue Zones"* was trademarked by Dan Buettner in November of 2005 in an article he wrote for the *National Geographic.* The article was about the lifestyles of the long-lived residents in Okinawa, Japan, Sardinia, the Nicoya Peninsula in Costa Rica, and Loma Linda, California. Aside from eating an anti-inflammatory diet or a Mediterranean diet, all of these people are physically active. All include walking as part of their fitness routines.

Walking offers the opportunity to connect with others. Your neighbors, your friends and family members would probably enjoy the chance to socialize and establish a routine for exercise. Look into walking clubs. There are opportunities to support various social causes through organized walks. This is a great way to broaden your support system and build a new circle of friends.

Overall, walking and exercise are important to add to your new approach to health. It supports your immune system that can then more effectively fight the inflammatory response that your body has been dealing with. The results will be profound. Walking reduces stress. Your mood will improve. From the extra activity and oxygen intake, you'll sleep better at night. Digestion improves. Walking fights the effects of weight producing hormones. It even reduces the risk for type 2 diabetes. Exercise and walking are important. Invest in this time.

Meditation

Anxiety and chronic stress trigger inflammation. To deal with uncomfortable feelings, the body sends inflammation markers to help cope with the experience. These markers release the stress hormone cortisol. Cortisol generates the harmful inflammation producing chemical, cytokine, that wreaks havoc on a person's immune system. The reaction to stress can lead to depression, sleepless nights, anxiety, over-eating, high blood pressure, and possibly turning to substances that appear to help us escape challenging realities. All of these are negative coping behaviors and reactions that are harmful to our health.

It is imperative, then, to learn how to cope with stress. We can't escape stress. It arrives to us in all kinds of forms. Good stress with a new job, a new baby, a move can still be challenging. And, of course, there is the bad stress.

Thousands of studies on meditation have shown that it benefits mental and physical health. These studies consistently show that diseases are managed better and even disappear, sleep is improved, stress is reduced, focus is improved, various addictions are better managed, pain management is controlled, and even relationships get better when meditation is practiced.

A study of over 2,400 individuals using mindful meditation showed a reduction in anxiety among those who suffered from a variety of mental health issues such as social anxiety, panic disorders, obsessive-compulsive disorders, and job-related anxiety. Another study of 4,600 subjects found long-term ease from depression.

A practice called "Mindful Meditation" has been proven to reduce the inflammatory response created by stress. One study showed that this type of meditation reduced the inflammatory response in 1,300 individuals. The people with the highest levels of stress were found to experience the greatest benefit.

Harvard has concurred with what yogis have been saying for thousands of years that with meditation we increase our emotional capacity for happiness, empathy, better moods, creativity, and viewing problems as smaller and more manageable.

The Journal of Biobehavioral Medicine published findings of a study of brain alterations consistent with mindful meditation practices. Over an 8-week clinical trial in a workplace setting that evaluated emotions of healthy employees, the findings from brain electrical activity were consistent with reports of increased positive emotions.

Meditation is strongly liked to improvements in physical health. Harvard's studies on meditation confirm that there are reductions in tension related pain such as pain associated with ulcers, muscle and joint pain, tension headaches and ulcers. A Wake Forest study on meditation confirmed in 2011that after only 4 days of mindful meditation their subjects experienced a reduction in pain by 57 percent and pain intensity was reduced by lessened by 40 percent.

The Mayo Clinic has reported results from their studies that support meditation's ability to manage such diseases as asthma, cancer, chronic pain syndromes, heart disease, high blood pressure, and irritable bowel syndrome. These are findings from October, 2017.

There is a large variety of meditation styles and practices. With so many types, there will surely be one that appeals to you.

Body Scan or Progressive Meditation

To do a body scan or progressive meditation you'll want to block out at least 20 to 30 minutes of time where you won't be interrupted. Find a place where you know you'll be left alone and not bothered by people's needs or duties hanging overhead. This is a time to get away from all of that.

As you begin, notice your body parts that come in contact with the chair you're sitting in or the mat on which you are sitting. Take a moment or two to make sure that you are as comfortable as you can make yourself. Even a little adjustment can make a difference to your ability to relax and let go of stress that you're experiencing in your body.

Imagine that you are taking a tour of your body. Start by noticing the feel of the clothes you're wearing. Notice the texture and weight of the blanket that might be covering you.

Move to your body parts. Don't visualize your body parts, just experience them. Just feel them. Focus on the sensations at the top of your head; your forehead; your ears; your eyebrows; your eyes; cheeks; lips. Just work your way down your body. You can also work from your toes on up. Notice the sensations in the soles of your feet; your ankles; your calves; knees; thighs and so on. After you scan a body part, allow that part to fade of from your consciousness.

If you have an instructor or are using an app, you'll probably be guided to connect body parts. You'll then connect your head to your neck. Then connect your neck to your torso. Finally, you'll be aware of wrapping your skin around your body.

There are variations on body scans. This is a simple explanation of how it goes. Body scans are helpful for people with chronic pain syndromes. It helps them to see that not all of their body is in pain. They can discover that parts of their body are pain free.

Yoga Nidra

Yoga nidra means "sleep with awareness." It's a relaxation practice intended to induce mental, emotional and physical relaxation. Some people report that a session of yoga nidra is as restorative of several hours of sleep.

There are differences between meditation and yoga nidra. In meditation, you are typically seated. You're comfortable, upright and alert. In the practice of yoga nidra, you are lying down.

In meditation, there is typically one anchor to hold your attention. It's often the breath. In a yoga nidra session, you are guided. Your attention is guided to specific places in a step by step manner.

In yoga nidra, you move into a state of deep conscious sleep. You're not in a waking state of consciousness, and you're past the dreaming state of consciousness. You are awake, but in the deep sleep state.

The benefits of yoga nidra are many, but not limited to reducing insomnia, decreasing anxiety, managing PTSD and chronic pain. It helps people recover from stress. Yoga nidra helps people recover from illness. It can assist in managing substance abuse.

The need for this restful practice in this frantic, high-tech world is more and more obvious. These are current statistics about sleep deprivation that people are experiencing.

~More than 30% of the general population is sleep deprived
~More than 60% of the over 60 population have insomnia
~More than 50% of Americans lose sleep due to anxiety and stress
~More than 10% of Americans use prescription sleep medicines and many more use over the counter sleep aids

The inflammation that is caused by stress and lack of sleep, as we know, causes a plethora of illnesses and diseases. Among them are mental health issues that can further exacerbate inflammation within the physical body. Yoga nidra is a meditation that can ease the tensions of modern life and provide a healing sleep experience.

Mindfulness Meditation

This is what mindfulness meditation looks like. People sit upright with their feet flat on the floor, eyes closed with their palms resting on their knees. They are sitting in a quiet room with an environment they have created. They are guided to focus on the present by paying attention to bodily sensations, thoughts and emotions. Special attention is given to the breath.

People who practice mindfulness meditation say that they think more clearly and experience less stress in their lives.

Suzanne Westbrook, a retiree from her position as internal medicine doctor at Harvard says that: "Our minds wander all the time, either reviewing the past or planning for the future. Mindfulness teaches you the skill of paying attention to the present by noticing when your mind wanders off. Come back to your breath. It's a place where we can rest and settle our minds." She said this when teaching an eight-week course about reducing stress.

When we can't relax our bodies and calm our minds, we are at much higher risk of stroke, heart disease and a host of other illnesses due to the inflammation that is incurred by stress. Ongoing stress produces cortisol in our bodies that is responsible for these diseases among others.

The mindfulness meditation technique isn't about changing ourselves from what we already are. Its purpose is to teach us to be unconditionally present and accepting of whatever is happening at the moment in our lives. Mindfulness meditation teaches that when we accept, we are more able to let go. We won't have conflict in our minds about controlling things that we can't control anyway. This reduces stress.

The philosophy argues that when we try to escape pain and cling to pleasure, the opposite effect takes place. The attempt to escape and control doesn't perpetuate our happiness. It causes us to suffer.

When we are mindful, we can show up for our lives. We're not experiencing our lives by wishing it was something a little different. We won't be able to live our lives to the fullest, and be present if we are worrying if something good will last or not.

Basically, the practice involves three things: body, breath and thoughts.

First create your environment. For many people, it's something as simple as lighting a candle or burning incense. This is to remind themselves of the impermanence of life. Other people make it more involved by decorating altars with flowers, pictures and objects from their own tradition.

Find a cushion or a chair to sit on. Make sure that you will be able to sit upright. Don't choose a chair that you know will give you back strain. Put your hands on your thighs and tilt your face downward. Your gaze is soft and resting on the floor.

Don't fight it when your mind wanders. It will wander. The point is to bring your mind back to your breath, your body and the environment that you've created.

The second part of the practice is to breathe. Just breathe. There is no special technique used. Paying attention to how you just are is what's supposed to be happening. Don't worry about controlling or manipulating the breath. Don't allow yourself to get caught up in what you're doing with your breathing.

The last part of the practice is working with your thoughts. People's minds wander. We have thoughts about the past, what's happening this afternoon. We'll have little fantasies. We might remember a favorite song from long ago. Thoughts can overlap and get jumbled. When this happens, gently, very gently bring your mind back to the breath. Don't be upset with yourself. This happens a lot, especially when you're just beginning to use this kind of meditation style. This meditation is not about making ourselves stop thinking. Becoming blank isn't the goal of most meditations. It certainly isn't part of a mindful meditation practice.

If this practice is new to you, try meditating for 10 minutes. Gradually, you'll build up to 20 to 30 minutes. If you've been doing this for some time, a 45-minute meditation will be a welcome routine. There is no judgment at all about how long you meditate. This meditation is about acceptance.

Zen Meditation

Zen meditation, also known as Zazen, is a meditation technique based from the Buddhist philosophy.

Practitioners typically begin by sitting in a Lotus position, sitting on a mat with legs crossed. The attention is focused inward. Some say that this is achieved by counting breaths, and others say no counting is done.

Zen meditation is about presence of mind. In Zen meditation, the practitioner's eyes are slightly open. In their minds, they gently steer away from any thoughts in an attempt to think about nothing. Once practitioners are able to keep their minds from wandering, the goal is to be able to tap into the unconscious mind. Once mastering this, you can become more cognizant of preconceived ideas and gain better understanding of yourself.

Loving Kindness Meditation

Some people call this a "radical act of love." As modern life seems to continue to accelerate creating stress and insecurity, more and more people are looking to this type of meditation as a method of self-care.

Of all the different meditation practices, loving kindness may be one of the best antidotes to fear and rage of our modern social experience. This practice is a non-reactive and non-judgmental way of addressing the anxiety provoking realities of our current society that are so inflammatory to our minds and our bodies.

How this works. Place yourself in a comfortable position. It can be lying down or you can be seated. Use the position that will work best for you. Let your breath relax you and allow you to be present. Let it flow.

Next, picture someone in your life who loves you or someone you love. Give yourself over to the emotions created by this relationship. Really tap into the feelings and emotions accorded to you by this person. Breathe into those feelings. Bathe in the experience that you are unconditionally accepted and loved just as you are by this person or these people.

You might have a feeling that you are not deserving or worthy of this strong love. That doesn't matter. It's irrelevant. What matters is that you are or were loved for who you are. Not what you might have been or what you once were. Allow yourself to drink in the feeling of love and allow yourself to be wrapped in these strong emotions.

Now, when you feel ready, see if you can become the source as well as the recipient of these feelings. Make these feelings your own so that you can give back these feelings of love and kindness and acceptance to others. Listen to your heartbeat. Rest and breathe in these feelings of absolute self-acceptance, love and forgiveness.

As you rest in this space of love and kindness for yourself, you can whisper a sort of mantra that will deepen this experience. They should be stated in the present tense, as if these things now exist. It could be something like: *I am safe. I am happy and content. I am healed and healthy.* Repeat one or two phrases like this at least three times. You may feel a little foolish when you begin this part of the practice, but in time you'll find that it's a part of what you truly feel about yourself. There will naturally be times when your mind wanders during this practice. But keep in mind that this isn't about judging yourself. Allow yourself to bring yourself back to the emotions of love and kindness. Be soft with yourself.

When learning about this practice, many people ask: "Why am I focusing so much on myself? This feels self-absorbed." The goal of this meditation is to help us recognize and feel that we are a part of this entire cosmos. We are no better and no less than anyone else. We belong and we have to include ourselves in this loving practice so that we can authentically share this love and acceptance with others without reservation.

The loving kindness is a kind of field of energy that can reach everyone, but it must begin with ourselves. It can be extended to people with whom you've had conflict, people who had been cruel to you. This is about love and forgiveness.

The anti-inflammatory lifestyle reflects old practices from long ago that will guide us as we go forward. Experiment with different types of meditation that will fit you. Adapt styles as you need to. Always keep in mind that there is no right or wrong way to meditate. The point of meditation is to reduce stress, to calm your mind and offer ease to your mind and emotions.

Practicing Gratitude

Practicing gratitude alters the way we respond to stress which improves cortisol levels. High cortisol levels amp up inflammation which needs to be eliminated or at least reduced. Gratitude gives us the ability to view our situation in a new way. Anxiety is managed over things we can't control. Practicing gratitude helps release us from cycles of worry that eventually damage our health.

Research studies on practicing gratitude have shown that gratitude strengthens relationships, makes people happier and improves health. It increases the ability to deal with stress. Gratitude balances hormones. Studies show that cultivating appreciation increases favorable changes in hormonal balance while decreasing the stress hormone, cortisol.

Thankfulness is felt on the biochemical level. It activates the frontal lobe of the brain when there is an emotional connection to the things you are grateful for. The hormones dopamine and serotonin are released and produce a sense of awe and comfort.

Practicing gratitude reduces cravings for more. When we are truly thankful, we don't feel a lack of abundance. We don't need more. We don't need more food, more fun, more activity and material things. Cravings are reduced so that we have a greater appreciation for people we love, the things we have, the food we eat, and the health that's given to us from these foods.

To reap the most benefit of this practice, make it a routine. Some people like to contemplate what they are thankful for at the beginning of the day. Others use this as a way to prepare for bed. A key part of this practice is to think of two or three things for which you are grateful, and spend time visualizing and reaching for the emotion that that person or thing gives to us. Gratitude enriches the mind-body connection by focusing on the emotions you generate as you practice thankfulness. Your heart is a center of energy. By practicing gratitude, you can open yourself to new experiences and feelings.

Keep a gratitude journal. Just by looking at it can elicit a feeling of calm as you review lists or written thoughts about what makes you thankful. Keep it in a place of easy access. Set it on a table by a favorite chair or by your bedside. If it's visible, you'll be more likely to pick it up and use it.

The journal doesn't have to have new items listed every day. It's okay to repeat things for which you are grateful as often as you want, as long as they're authentic. You can be grateful many times for that daughter, son, significant other, parent, job or pet. Maybe you're grateful that your car hasn't had any problems. You could be thankful for the garden you planted. You can be grateful for clean water and air, electricity or that you have a roof over your head. The list is truly endless. One of your entry items could be about yourself. Don't leave yourself off this list! Don't overlook yourself. Think about all the things you've accomplished, even the small things. Celebrate yourself a little. You deserve it.

When we focus on what we presently have, it helps us stay in the here and now. We're not worrying about what we had in the past or might not have in the future. We're here, right now. Being present affects how we see life. When we're present, we enjoy it more. We can take the time to savor the food we eat. We look at the sky and the trees. We can smell the breezes and admire the fragrances of flowers. We find we're paying attention a little more. We can really see those people who mean so much to us.

Gratitude is a very attractive trait and it's contagious. You'll be saying, "Thank you" more often and you'll really mean it. You may find that after a time, that you're attracting more friends. And it's likely that they'll be people who share the same values as yourself.

Get Back to Nature

Even just a generation or two, everybody spent more time in natural surroundings than they do now. Because of that, people experience more stress and anxiety in big cities as well as in small towns. There are current bodies of work done by psychologists that report that there is an on-going spike in mental health illnesses such as depression and anxiety. We've spoken of how meditation can improve mood and calm nerves, thereby reducing the body's inflammation. But we haven't yet talked about how getting "back to nature" can soothe our psyches.

A graduate student named Gary Bratman has been studying the psychological effects of people living in urban areas against those who spend time in natural settings. In a study that he and his colleagues wrote while at Emmett Interdisciplinary Program in Environment and Resources at Stanford University they found that volunteers who strolled through the abundantly green campus were happier and alert than volunteers who spent the comparable amount of time walking by heavy multi-lane traffic. From that study, Mr. Bratman and his peers published an article in *Proceedings of the National Academy of Sciences* about levels of brain activity in the subgenual prefrontal cortex of all volunteers. It was found, not surprisingly, that the test subjects who walked amid the lush, green campus showed improvements in their overall mental health. The study showed that brain activity was less agitated. They brooded less and were happier.

It was concluded that the findings "strongly suggest that getting out into natural environments" could be an easy and effective way for those living in urban settings to relax and improve their moods.

Now, some of you might be thinking that a scientific study doesn't need to take place in order to get the same results. Most of us find that when up in the mountains, by a lake or the sea, spending any time in any natural setting enhances our well-being. Time with "Mother Nature" does so much for us and we wonder why we don't do it more often.

Our attitudes and mood improve. Our memories are sharper. Loneliness is reduced. The scents of the forest soothe our nerves. It's basically aromatherapy! We sleep better after taking time to be outside. Being outside improves our quality of life.

Nature Walks

There is now more information than ever before on the benefits of Nature Walks. There is a growing body of literature about the mental and physical advantages of
spending time walking in the outdoors. Recent research is even showing positive results of test subjects taking a "short micro-break" by taking some time to look at a nature scene. It's been shown that these rejuvenating moments have a positive effect on the adult brain resulting in greater attention spans. And for children, it gives them the ability to score higher on cognitive tests.

There have been numerous recent studies that point to the findings of reduced stress, better cardio-vascular health, healthy weight, stronger bones and cartilage, improved self-esteem and mood, and increased creative thinking. Walking outdoors makes people happier than working out in a gym.

The cellular activity that's been associated with nature walks through forests in particular have indicated possible links to production of anti-cancer proteins. The levels of these proteins have been found to last up to 7 days after a stroll through the forest. Studies from Japan, have discovered that in regions with large areas of forest that there are lower mortality rates from cancer even after considering cigarette smoking and lower socioeconomic status of the test subjects.

Nature walks have been proven to lower blood pressure. Research has confirmed that there is weight loss associated with walking outside. Nature walks help stave off colds and flu. It's been proven that our brains work better. The vitamin D we get from being outside and in sunlight reduces inflammation. Time in nature can improve longevity.

In children it's been demonstrated that spending time outdoors can protect their eyesight. The risk of developing nearsightedness (myopia) is greatly reduced. A 2012 review of this research concurred with those findings.

The objective of taking a nature walk doesn't have to be anything more than taking a break and enjoying the outdoors. However, there are a lot of things you can do to enhance the experience when the walk feels like it's becoming a little too routine. Here are some before, during and after activities that might bring the experience into a sharper focus.

~Focus in on the five senses. Pay marked attention to what you see, what you feel, what you taste, what you hear and smell and describe these things to yourself or your walking partner.
~Walk at different times of the day or evening. You might notice things that you hadn't before during your regular walking time.
~Sketch a picture of what you see. Skip taking pictures and selfies.
~Lay on a blanket and look up into the trees or the sky. Make cloud "pictures."
~Go barefoot and feel the grass, the dirt, the sand, and the water on your feet.
~Catch fireflies in the evening and let them go. It might bring back a lovely childhood memory.
~Collect fall leaves. Use them for a project at home.

~Paint rocks you find. Make people and houses or things you saw on your walk.
~Keep a journal about your walks.
~Listen to the birds, the air, the water.

John Muir said, "In every walk with Nature, one receives far more than he seeks." We all know this to be true. Nature walks are lovely opportunities for making discoveries, being creative, for getting relaxed, and just to enjoy ourselves. Taking the time to give ourselves this gift is a treasure.

Chapter 8: Two Week Diet Plan

The anti-inflammatory diet should contain pre-biotics, omega-3s, fiber, protein, healthy fats, vitamins, minerals and anti-oxidants. The meals should include whole grains, fatty fish, legumes, fresh fruit and vegetables. Remember to drink eight 8-ounces glasses of water daily, and only a moderate amount of red wine if allowed by your doctor. Keep in mind that it's a plant-based diet, with little or no red meat. Here is a place to start to get into the habit to cook foods that will feed your body and reduce your inflammation. The following meal plan ideas require little preparation and can be altered for convenience.

Week 1

Breakfast Choices:
~Oatmeal with berries and Greek Yogurt
~Raspberry/Strawberry/Blueberry Smoothie
~Buckwheat Pancakes with Berries)
~Granola, with Berries and Greek Yogurt
~Quinoa with Riced Cauliflower and Cinnamon
~Poached Salmon, Avocado and Poached Egg on Multi-grain Toast
~Muesli with Raspberries and Greek Yogurt

Lunch Choices:
~Avocado, Hummus and Radish Sandwich on Sprouted Bread
~Crushed Kale Salad, Red Onions and Mushrooms with Multi-grain Bread*
~Lemon/Garlic Zoodles and Green Salad
~Black Eyed Peas with Beets and Hazelnut Salad and Pita Bread*
~Color Bowl Salad Made with Vegetables with Color and Quinoa
~Stir Fried Tofu with Broccoli and Shredded Carrot
~Roasted Root Vegetables, Quinoa and Feta Salad

Dinner Choices:

~Curried Potatoes with Egg
~Salmon Cakes with Dark, Green Vegetable and Tomato Juice
~Vegetarian Chili
~Chicken Breast with Sweet Potatoes and Spinach and Basil
Salad
~Pan Fried Trout, Broccoli and Quinoa, Small Glass of Red
Wine
~Lentil and Chicken Soup with Sweet Potato and Spinach*
~Walnut Crusted Baked Salmon, Black Rice, Balsamic and
Parmesan Brussels Sprouts*

Snack Choices:
~Tart, red cherries
~Handful of Almonds with a Small Cup of Cantaloupe
~Plain Greek Yogurt with Berries
~Cottage Cheese with Walnuts and Cinnamon
~Sliced Tomato with Olives
~Small Handful of Dark Chocolate Chips and Walnuts

Week 2:

Breakfast Choices:
~Scrambled Eggs with Turmeric and Multigrain Toast
~Whole Grain English Muffin Topped with Ricotta, Almonds and
Honey
~Oatmeal with Cinnamon, Dates, Honey and Greek Yogurt*
~Two Slices of Whole Grain Toast with Ricotta Cheese and
Chopped Berries
~Baked Eggs with Avocado and Feta Cheese*
~Whole Wheat Pancakes Topped with Ricotta and Berries
~Pan Fried Egg with Multi-grain Toast, Tomatoes and
Avocados

Lunch Choices:
~Grilled Eggplant, Zucchini and Onion on Whole Wheat Toast
~Egg Frittata with Asparagus and Green Tossed Salad
~Mixed Salad Greens with Olives and Cherry Tomatoes

~*Roasted Spicy Anchovies with Avocados, Sprouts on Multi-grain Toast*
~*Bell Peppers, Olives, Sun-dried Tomatoes and Spinach on Quinoa**
~*Roasted Vegetables in Pita Pockets with Hummus*
~*White Bean Soup with Chicken, Raw Vegetable Slices*

Dinner Choices:
~*Arugula and Spinach Salad with Zucchini, Cherry Tomatoes, Boiled Egg and Sprouts with Pita Pocket and Hummus*
~*Whole Grain Pasta with Sun-dried Tomatoes, Grilled Vegetables and Rosemary, Small Glass of Red Wine*
~*Grilled Trout, Baked Sweet Potato and Green Salad*
~*Zoodle Spaghetti with Basil Pesto and Sliced Tomatoes*
~*Pita Pocket Topped with Feta, Steamed Spinach, Sun-dried Tomatoes and Kalamata Olives*
~*Grilled Tuna Steak with Baked Potato and Chives*
~*Roast Chicken with Turmeric, Wild Rice and Mint, Tossed Green Salad**

Snack Choices:
~*Two Plums and Almonds*
~*Handful of Dried Fruit*
~*Red Grapes and Walnuts*
~*Hard Cheese and Strawberries*
~*Plain Greek Yogurt with Drizzle of Honey*
~*Red Bell Pepper with Guacamole, Small Glass of Red Wine*
~*Apple Slices with Peanut Butter*

Recipes

Breakfast:

Poached Salmon, Avocado and Poached Egg on Multi-grain Toast

Ingredients:

½ C. dry white wine
½ C. water
2 lbs. salmon filets cut into 4 pieces
4 eggs
1 T. extra virgin olive oil
¼ tsp. freshly grated garlic
1 tsp. dried parsley
2 avocados sliced
Basil leaves
6 slices of multi-grain toast
Sea salt and pepper to taste

Bring the wine and water to a boil in a large pan. Add the salmon and spices into the wine and water, reduce heat to a simmer on medium heat. The salmon should be firm but tender after 10 minutes.

To poach the eggs, bring water to a simmer on medium heat in a medium-sized pan. Crack eggs, one by one, into the water and cook for 2 minutes. Remove the pan from the heat and let it sit for 8-10 minutes.

With a slotted spoon, lift eggs out of the water and let drain on a towel for a couple of minutes.

On each slice of warm multi-grain toast, place the salmon, the basil leaves and an egg on top. Garnish with avocado slices.

Serves 4.

Oatmeal with Cinnamon, Dates, Honey and Greek Yogurt

Ingredients:

1 C. Traditional breakfast oats
¼ C. dates
Honey and cinnamon to taste
½ C. Greek yogurt for each serving

Bring 1 ¾ C. water to a boil. Add the oats and stir for 1 minute as water continues to boil. Remove from heat, cover and let water absorb for 10 minutes.

Serve with dates, honey and cinnamon to taste with ½ C. Greek yogurt.

Serves 2.

Baked Eggs with Avocado and Feta Cheese

Ingredients:

3 T. extra virgin olive oil
1 small red onion chopped
1 clove garlic finely minced
½ jalapeno pepper finely minced, with seeds discarded
1 T. oregano
1 tsp. chili pepper
1 tsp. paprika
Fresh basil leaves
Sea salt and pepper to taste
6 eggs
1 avocado sliced
½ C. feta cheese

Preheat oven to 400 degrees F.

In a large cast iron skillet or other heavy cookware, saute the small red onion, the jalapeno and garlic in olive oil until the onion just begins to turn brown. Add spices and continue to saute for another 2 minutes.

Crack eggs into the onion mixture that has been spread evenly in the pan. If you don't have cast iron, you can transfer the mixture into a 9 x 13" pan that has been prepped with a light coating of olive oil.

Bake for 15-18 minutes. Garnish with avocado slices and basil leaves.

Serves 4 to 6.

Lunch:

Crushed Kale Salad, Red Onions and Mushrooms with Multi-grain Bread

Ingredients:

1 bunch kale
1 medium red onion sliced
¾ lb. sliced white mushrooms

Dressing:
¼ C. balsamic vinegar
½ C. extra virgin olive oil
½ tsp. thyme

Saute red onions in 2 T. extra virgin olive oil on medium heat. In another pan, saute mushrooms in 2 T. extra virgin olive oil on medium heat, as well.
Rinse and dry kale. Crush in your hands before tearing (it makes it sweeter).

Combine the onion, the mushrooms and kale and toss. Top with dressing.

Dressing: Combine the balsamic vinegar, the oil and the thyme and stir or shake.

Serves 4.

Bell Peppers, Olives, Sun-dried Tomatoes and Spinach on Quinoa

Ingredients:

1 bell pepper sliced
½ C. sliced Kalamata olives
½ C. sun-dried tomatoes
2 C. fresh spinach
2 C. cooked quinoa
2 T. extra virgin olive oil

Prepare quinoa as directed on package. Rinse and dry spinach. Saute the sliced bell pepper in olive oil until tender and add olives just at the end.

Arrange the cooked bell peppers, olives and sun-dried tomatoes on bed of quinoa.

Black Eyed Peas with Beets and Hazelnut Salad and Pita Bread

Ingredients:

1 15 oz. can of black-eyed peas rinsed
1 C. cooked shredded beets (canned or fresh)
½ C. chopped hazelnuts

Dressing:
¼ C. balsamic vinegar
½ C. extra virgin olive oil
1 tsp. thyme

Rinse the black-eyed peas. Place in individual bowls. Top with beets, chopped hazelnuts and dressing.

Serves 2.

Dinner:

Walnut Encrusted Salmon

Ingredients:
1 lb. salmon cut in half
¼ C. breadcrumbs
¼ C. walnuts
1 T. dijon mustard
½ tsp. cayenne pepper
2 T. honey

Preheat oven to 375 degrees F.

Grind walnuts in small food processor. Mix well with honey, mustard, and cayenne pepper and spread onto salmon. Bake at 375 degrees F for 20 minutes.

Serves 2.

Roast Chicken with Turmeric

Ingredients:
1 3-4 lb. whole chicken
1 head garlic

¼ C. extra virgin olive oil
2 tsp. sea salt
2 tsp. turmeric
1 tsp. black pepper

Preheat oven to 375 degrees F.

Rinse and dry chicken and place in roasting pan. Rub the chicken with olive oil. Mix the salt, turmeric and black pepper together and sprinkle this over the top of the chicken, and rub some in the cavity.

Cut the head of garlic in half crosswise. Place garlic in pan with the cut side facing down.

Roast for 1 hour and check for doneness. If the flesh is pink near the bone, it will require more time. It can be covered while roasting to prevent drying out and burning the skin. It should be golden brown when finished.

Serves 4 to 6.

Lentil and Chicken Soup with Sweet Potato and Spinach

Ingredients:
3 T. extra virgin olive oil
1 medium onion chopped
2-3 cloves garlic minced
2 carrots chopped
½ tsp. cayenne
1 tsp. turmeric
1 tsp. cumin
1 ½ freshly grated ginger
4 C. low sodium chicken broth
1 15 oz. can coconut milk
1 C. lentils
3 C. shredded chicken breast

Sea salt and black pepper to taste
Garnish: Sprigs of fresh cilantro

Saute onion in olive oil on low heat for 5 minutes, stirring occasionally. Then add garlic and spices, carrots and ginger continuing to saute for another 2 minutes.

Add the chicken broth, and lentils and cook until lentils are tender. You may need to add water to the broth.

Add coconut milk and cook until soup thickens. Taste and adjust seasoning to taste. Garnish with cilantro.

Serves 4 to 6.

Conclusion

Lifestyle choices can help you live your best life. Of course, no one herb or one food will stave off a disease. Your health is determined by genetics, your diet and your lifestyle. By utilizing a program with a diet that is guided by principles of anti-inflammatory eating, exercising, getting enough sleep and reducing stress you'll be able to attain goals that will prevent or reduce sickness and give you a brighter outlook. Within a short amount of time, the disciplines written about in this book will become second nature. You will have mastered the tools to allow you to live a healthy, rich and rewarding life. Enjoy!

www.ingramcontent.com/pod-product-compliance
Lightning Source LLC
Chambersburg PA
CBHW051030030426
42336CB00015B/2805